LOVE NEVER ENDS

Wife of a Cornish farmer, mother to two young daughters, Jenny Richards lived a full life. Then Motor Neurone Disease struck.

By the time her book was finished, Jenny was unable to walk, to speak or to swallow food. The illness had made a ruthless advance through her physical abilities.

She was not expected to live much longer, yet she writes, 'I feel completely normal inside. My mind still teems with ideas. My spirit still dances.'

What is it like for a spirit richly alive to be trapped in a failing body? How can she cope physically? Can her faith carry her through? How are her husband and children affected?

Jenny Richards' story was featured in *Family Circle*'s Winning Through series.

The Duchess of York, Patroness of the Motor Neurone Disease Association, has contributed a foreword to the book. She speaks from personal acquaintance with this remarkable woman who 'has communicated her special light to the world'.

This book is dedicated to:

Anthony: for his strength, patience and unquenchable hopefulness;

Claire: for her sensitivity and 'motherly' protectiveness;

Rebecca: for her resilience and sense of fun;

All our family and friends through whom the tidal wave of God's love flows;

And to the memory of my Mum and Dad who taught me the joy of family life

Love Never Ends

Jenny Richards

A LION PAPERBACK
Oxford · Batavia · Sydney

Copyright © 1990 Jenny Richards

Published by
Lion Publishing plc
Sandy Lane West, Oxford, England
ISBN 0 7459 1962 6
Lion Publishing Corporation
1705 Hubbard Avenue, Batavia, Illinois 60510, USA
ISBN 0 7459 1962 6
Albatross Books Pty Ltd
PO Box 320, Sutherland, NSW 2232, Australia
ISBN 0 7324 0260 3

First edition 1990

British Library Cataloguing in Publication Data
Richards, Jenny
Love never ends.
1. Man. Nervous system. Motor neurone disease
2. Title
616.8
ISBN 0 7459 1962 6

Printed and bound in Great Britain
by Cox and Wyman Ltd, Reading

For further information about Motor Neurone Disease contact:

Motor Neurone Disease Association, P.O. Box 246, Northampton, NN1 1TR; tel: 0800 626262

A.L.S. Association, 15300 Ventura Boulevard, Suite 315, Sherman Oaks, CA 91403; tel: (818) 990 2151

A.L.S. Society, Suite 24, 2nd Floor, 2 Holden Street, Ashfield, NSW 2131; tel: (02) 799 8519

Motor Neurone Society, C.P.O. Box 397, Auckland; tel: (09) 410 4034

CONTENTS

PREFACE

In 1987, at the age of thirty-three, I was a fairly typical overworked, underpaid farmer's wife and mother of two small children! Into a week I crammed the usual cleaning, tidying and cooking, plus part-time teaching, Sunday-school teaching, a little preaching, playgroup duties and occasional care of foster children. Life was hectic but good. I felt 'in control' and was looking forward to a developing teaching career as the children became more independent. The future looked rosy.

In this book I want to relate how an illness virtually wiped out this pattern of living and dashed all my plans and aspirations. How gradually, after much frustration, anger and disappointment, God's love filled the void and started giving me new goals and a new purpose in life.

Jenny

Chapter 1
DEATH SENTENCE

On Friday 27 May 1988, I wrote a lengthy entry in my diary. I think it best expresses how I felt that bright, early-summer morning when the men were cutting silage in the fields and the campions and bluebells were more vibrant than ever in the country lanes around our farm:

> *'It's a strange feeling I have today. I'm in that state of shock one feels when a loved one dies, only there is no business to attend to...*
>
> *At 9.30 this morning Anthony and I were informed by a kindly specialist that I have a terminal disease— Motor Neurone Disease, they call it. My speech and ability to swallow will deteriorate. I have less than two years to live...*
>
> *I'm not feeling sorry for myself particularly. I'm not afraid of death—not the state of being dead, just a little fearful of dying. My worst fears are those for Anthony and the children. Claire is six, Rebecca almost four. I don't want to leave them. I want to see what they 'do', who they marry, their children...*
>
> *The specialist has arranged for me to go to a London hospital to have the diagnosis confirmed. This is primarily for our peace of mind, not because of doubts on his part.*
>
> *I'm a Christian but I'm not sure how I feel about*

healing. I always thought that it works for other people but not for me, but then I always thought other people had terminal illnesses. I've asked our Minister to call tomorrow and I've been invited to a healing service at the Baptist Church at Falmouth—right opposite the house where I was born. Perhaps I should go...

The silly thing is that, despite my death sentence, I feel no different, physically, today than yesterday. I must obviously live one day at a time.

This afternoon I'll go for a walk with Rebecca and my next-door neighbour, Jo...'

The past few months had certainly been bleak. Christmas had come to an abrupt end when, on Boxing Day, my father died suddenly as I took him an early morning cup of tea. This in itself was devastating. Although seventy-four, he was an extremely active Christian man, preaching every Sunday and making numerous pastoral visits during the week. As an only child I had been extremely close to both my parents and was still grieving over my mother's premature death ten years previously. She died just after Anthony and I became engaged and I desperately missed her love and friendship.

With both parents wrenched away I felt bereft. I had tried to maintain the stiff British upper lip and to immerse myself in busyness but, as the bleak January days faded into even bleaker February days, I felt darker and darker inside and my emotions became unsteadier by the day. There were days when I couldn't stop crying and I hated myself for being so weak.

At the same time I began to slur my speech—very embarrassing for a virtual teetotaller—and had difficulty in swallowing. 'It's shock!' everyone assured me, but it worsened until, in March, I had to see the doctor. He referred me to the neurologist who, after various scans, delivered the grim diagnosis in May.

Motor Neurone Disease is a disease of the nervous system which renders muscles useless. For some people it starts in the limbs, but for others, like me, it firstly affects the muscles used for speech and eating and swallowing food. It also affects the emotions and there is often a thin line between uncontrollable crying and unreasonable laughter. At the time of writing there is no proven treatment and the best that specialists can offer is to put patients in touch with support groups and various therapists.

So there I was on 27 May 1988 with all my plans for the future crumbling around me. How could God possibly salvage me and my family from such devastation?

Chapter 2
CARRIED BY FRIENDS

There is a marvellous account in the gospels about the healing of a paralyzed man. It is a story which has become very significant to our family during the past year. The paralyzed man needed healing, but there was no way in which he could reach Jesus by himself, so he was carried on a makeshift bed to the house where Jesus was preaching. We are told in Luke's gospel that 'they tried to take him into the house and put him in front of Jesus. Because of the crowd, however, they could find no way to take him in. So they carried him up on the roof, made an opening in the tiles, and let him down on his bed into the middle of the group in front of Jesus.' What determination these people had, and what great friends they were. How they were rewarded! For we read that Jesus recognized their great faith, and healed the man. On many occasions we have been in the position of this paralyzed man: we have run out of strength, almost too weary in mind, body and spirit to pray. Yet, always, at those lowest moments, friends have phoned, written or called with the right words of encouragement, practical help or a prayer. We have indeed been often carried by friends.

It was these friends who whirled into action within hours of the diagnosis. Their individual reactions are etched on my mind, each one a cameo of God's love in action.

One of the first to call was Mary—a cousin's wife and one of the close farming community in our area. Mary is down-to-earth, capable and practical, everyone's mother. We talked and cried together. In Mary, Jesus' compassion flowed and I felt the warmth of his love for me at that very moment.

My father-in-law was next. He is a quiet, deeply spiritual man with a lovely sense of humour. Since my own father's death he had become even more special to me. Then, as on many subsequent occasions, we stood in the middle of the breakfast room, arms linked, while he quietly and quite naturally prayed out loud for me, and with me. He seemed to lift me up to God as he prayed. Although only a small man physically, his words and prayers made me feel safe and strong.

Then Lynn stormed in. We had been close friends since the age of twelve, and it was at her wedding that Anthony and I met. Both of us were 'only' children, and we had become like sisters. Lynn was furious. 'I've been telling God that he's got his wires crossed,' she said. 'All the way over in the car I've been shouting at him!' Lynn continued to bring determination and cheerfulness to our situation. She was always there with a listening ear, a box of tissues and constructive help. Immediately she organized armies of people to pray. By the following Sunday, people in churches the length and breadth of Britain were remembering us in their prayers.

On the following morning, the minister of our church, Derek Polgreen, came. This visit, and all the ones that followed, was unhurried and full of calm and patient understanding. He always brought with him the aroma of God's peace, and a great deal of encouragement. He was the first to pray with us for healing. There were no bells or flashing lights, but with quiet confidence we looked to God.

'Love gifts'—gifts of food or things we might need— were to be a regular feature of our lives and a very tangible sign of God's love to us, shown through friends. In the kitchen I usually have a little pile of trays, bowls or flan cases which have contained pasties, cakes or pies made for us by other people. That first weekend we received a beautiful flower arrangement from the play-group of which I was chairman, and pies and sponges from various friends.

It was through all this loving support that on the Saturday evening I could write in my diary:

> *'I know we are all in God's hands, even though the way is puzzling and uncertain at the moment... There will be lots of people praying for us tomorrow. I know I've got to let go and be immersed in God's will for me.'*

The 'letting go' was not always easy. As human beings we like to be in control and to feel that we can sort out our own problems. Yet Jesus hands out an invitation to each of us: 'Come to me, all of you who are tired from carrying heavy loads, and I will give you rest.' Why are we so slow to claim that 'rest'?

That first Sunday after the diagnosis was to be an exciting day and the beginning of an extraordinary spiritual journey for Anthony and me. We both came from a Methodist background and attended the small village chapel of Frogpool where I taught in the Sunday School and Anthony is the Treasurer. I had made a personal commitment to Jesus when I was fourteen at a Methodist Youth Conference. Anthony had never made such a commitment and, although a stalwart of the chapel, confessed to being rather uncertain about the personal relevance of Christianity. Yet, from the moment my illness was named, Anthony began to blossom spiritually. He increasingly displayed God-given strength and wisdom. In fact, he was being led into a new spiritual dimension.

I couldn't face our close little congregation that

Sunday morning, so Anthony and the children went along. This was not altogether easy for Anthony. Some well-meaning people offered sympathetic noises in the form of, 'Whatever will you do? How are you going to manage?' While the praying nucleus were asking God for healing, others had already buried me!

That dinner-time I struggled with my meal and couldn't make any headway at all to swallow the roast lamb. All I could hear drumming in my head were the words, 'Your swallowing and speech will deteriorate... two years at the most.'

Another friend, Chris Ryall, took us in her car that Sunday evening to Falmouth Baptist Church. That evening's service was billed as a healing service, but the greatest immediate impact was the sense of freedom and excitement in the way everybody was worshipping God, both in the music and in the prayers. After the previous two days spent imploring God to help me, this was a refreshing change and the start of a vital lesson for me: when we praise God we are looking away from ourselves and our problems and opening up a channel through which God can heal.

At the end of the service the pastor invited people to come forward for prayer. Such open ministry was not part of my Methodist background and I wasn't sure what to expect. With trepidation I made my way to the front. The pastor and his wife prayed with me, and then another new experience—the pastor began to pray in a beautiful unknown language. This was the 'gift of tongues' mentioned in the New Testament which, until that time, I had never heard used. Although new, it didn't frighten me because the love of God was so obviously flowing through the words. His wife interpreted: 'God says he loves you very much... he has not forgotten you.'

As I returned to my seat, Anthony and I experienced a great sense of peace. Was I healed? There was no

13

improvement in my speech, but when I tackled some cold meat and salad for my supper, it didn't take me long to polish off the lot! God had confirmed his love to me by this sign of physical improvement. Was it possible that I could receive complete physical healing?

We had hurriedly arranged a few days' holiday in Gloucester during the school half-term. An aunt and uncle lived near there and my cousin, Penny, and her two children were also within reach. Before we set off Anthony thrust the Bible in front of me and read part of Psalm 130. It was to be the first of many 'given' verses.

> 'I rely on your constant love
> I will be glad, because you will rescue me.
> I will sing to you, O Lord,
> Because you have been good to me.'

So, on Monday morning, we set off—both on holiday and on our uncertain future—with a note of praise in our hearts and on our lips.

Chapter 3
WHY?

It was not an easy holiday for any of us. We were still reeling from the shock of the diagnosis, and my emotions were in turmoil. We might be pursuing quite ordinary holiday pursuits, such as wandering round the wildfowl park or a butterfly garden, and suddenly the realization of what was happening to me would descend like a heavy, black cloud. Whenever the children said something touching or did something amusing it would make me hurt deep inside because I loved them so much and couldn't bear the thought of leaving them. Then, to my horror, a really ugly emotion surfaced—jealousy.

We were enjoying our time with my cousin Penny and her daughter, Georgina. It was Georgina's twelfth birthday and I was making a real effort to keep cheerful and not spoil her day. We were sitting around after lunch, drinking coffee and discussing my Uncle and Aunty's plans to move further west to Plymouth—only an hour or so away from where we live. Suddenly I felt as if I could see a future emerging in which I had no part. Everybody would be happy except for me. Perhaps once Uncle and Aunty had moved, Penny would as well. They would share experiences with my family that would be denied me. That was it—God wanted me out of the way so that everyone else could be happy. I suddenly felt jealous of all the people in this imaginary future.

Despite all positive acts and words of love I had already experienced, and despite knowing that I could trust God for the future, here was I letting negative thoughts infiltrate my mind. It was a lesson I had to learn—to transform those negative thoughts into positive ones and to experience the difference it makes.

Then, a few days later, we were wandering round Bristol Zoo and I found myself looking at other families, especially the mums, and envying them their health. 'It's all right for them,' I kept thinking, 'they aren't going to die and leave two lovely children.' These dreadful feelings of jealousy only lasted two or three weeks but, while they did, they were a nightmare in themselves. I felt they were so unlovely that I couldn't admit them to anyone, not even Anthony, and I felt so guilty.

Anger was another powerful emotion. I was angry with God for knocking me down just as I was 'getting on my feet.' My Mum had died just over ten years ago, in October 1977. At the time I had made a mammoth effort to 'keep going', mainly to support my Dad. We had a sort of unspoken pact that we would go on bravely with our normal activities and so I was preaching again the week after Mum died and six weeks later I helped Dad plough through the endless Christmas card list. All the time I was pushing my hurt, bitterness and anger deep under the surface. Now I would dispute the wisdom of this 'British' bravery. Now I understand much more what it means to say that Jesus died for our griefs and sorrows as well as for our sins. I should have taken time to open up my innermost being to him and let his love flow in and heal my wounds.

A year after Mum died, and four months before Anthony and I were due to be married, my Dad's diabetes became extremely bad and he was in hospital for the whole of December and January. During this time I was told he was unlikely to pull through. When he did emerge from hospital he was very weak, and it was this pale figure who accompanied me down the aisle on 7 April 1979. I had been greatly helped in the wedding arrangements by my friend Lynn, and her parents, but I was so missing my Mum's companionship and enthusiastic involvement. Like most mothers and daughters we had often mused about the Wedding Day and she had developed a great fondness for Anthony, as he had for her. Brides, however, have to be radiant and cheerful and I felt I mustn't let the image slip, and so the hurting was pushed still deeper.

I then threw my energies into the early months of marriage, while still trying to keep an eye on Dad and travelling quite a distance each day to the school where I taught English. It was during this time that I started being dogged by what the doctors labelled 'nervous attacks'. I would feel extremely light in the head and very uncomfortable about sitting in one place for any length of time in case the dizziness started. Sometimes, also, as I walked, the ground would appear to rise and fall under my feet. I believe now it was due to the suppressed tensions and hurts erupting like miniature volcanoes from deep within... I needed inner healing.

So many exciting and wonderful things happened in our first eight years of marriage—the birth of our two daughters, the acquisition of our own farm and the subsequent move to a large and lovely farmhouse, even if it did shriek out for redecoration throughout! Of course buying the farm meant that our expenditure had to be kept to a minimum—enough to cover bills, but not enough to save for a rainy day, a holiday or the dreaded expense of Christmas. In fact this used to worry me a great deal so, like many mums, I embarked on a couple of projects to make a little extra money, without having to leave the home.

One of these schemes was to join forces with my neighbour, Jo, and produce p4asties for a few local shops. These became quite successful and we found our kitchens almost permanently under siege from pastry, flour, onions, and so on. Eventually we closed down the production line and switched to Celebration cakes. This was good fun and even led to an interview on our local radio station, although I've always maintained they were probably hard up for material, as it was bad weather.

Also I started some child-minding. Besides providing extra income, it gave Rebecca some company after Claire started school. This led to an interesting contact with the Social Services who wanted to know if we were interested in a Family Support Scheme. In our case it entailed looking after two little boys for occasional weekends while their foster parents had a break. So it was we met Nigel and Roger. Nigel was seven. He had a severe kidney complaint, but his greatest problems were due to emotional scars. Whenever he visited he became very possessive in relation to me and, to begin with, Claire found it particularly difficult. Nigel taught us all a great deal about patience, and forbearance. He had some irritating and amusing ways such as insisting on calling Anthony 'Nantony' and always looking at every meal and saying 'I don't eat that!' although we knew he had wolfed the lot on his last visit.

Roger was three and suffered cerebral palsy. During his time with us he was in an exciting period of development. It was discovered that, although he was unable to communicate, he understood a great deal, and various people were working hard to increase his mobility, and even to move him on to using a computer. He used to whizz around the house in a little battery-run chair, looking like a little robot. It was very rewarding to care for Roger and see him developing so quickly. In fact I began to consider teaching children with special needs. But that would have meant attending a residential course which was obviously not practical.

During this period the 'dizzy' problems were lessening and I was growing in confidence again, so when I saw an advertisement for a part-time teacher at a nearby village school I didn't hesitate to apply. The post was to teach top Juniors for one-and-a-half days a week while the headmaster attended to administrative duties. Naturally, I prayed about applying for the job, asking God to guide me. Before I went for the interview I remember feeling very peaceful. I felt that this was where God wanted me. I did get the job and thoroughly enjoyed almost every moment. Previously I had taught eleven- to sixteen-year-olds, and I found the enthusiasm of these nine- and ten-year-olds very refreshing. Also I enjoyed going into a different environment for part of the week. The head teacher was encouraging and said he foresaw a time when I could apply for a full-time post. The money I earned boosted our overall earnings by fifty per cent. For the first time in six years I wasn't worrying about our money. Everything seemed to be improving...and then, the blow!

Why was it, I asked God, that he had knocked me down like this? I felt like a skittle, set up just to be walloped over again. Yes, I was angry with God. One Sunday morning I decided to find an open space and shout at him. I put on my wellies and squelched up the lane to a square in front of the silage store. With my failing voice I 'socked' it to God. Then I stumped back down the lane again. Perhaps I should have stopped to listen for a reply...?

In all the ups and downs—especially the downs—God continued to use friends to bring me his encouragement. We had been to the Royal Cornwall Show—the annual agricultural 'feast' for farmers. Our visit this year had been depressing for two reasons. Firstly the Motor Neurone Disease Society had a tent where they were making people aware of the disease and asking for support to finance research. It was positioned just off the main ring and, while the children delighted in watching the horses, with brasses gleaming, prance around the ring, all I could see was a huge, bleak poster declaring, 'Motor Neurone Disease paralyzes.' We had also arranged to meet a counsellor there—this didn't improve my mood. I knew she was trying to be helpful, but being told not to bother about house renovation, just to concentrate on doing the things we've always wanted, didn't do much for morale! Part of me didn't want to face the inevitable outcome of the disease.

Secondly my feelings of jealousy surfaced again. We had met up with Anthony's cousin Philip and his wife, Mary. As we walked around the rabbit tent and then went to look at the poultry and sheep, Mary chatted enthusiastically to the children and they were obviously enjoying her company. I could no longer speak to my children in such a free and easy way: I had to limit my failing speech to commands or 'forbids'. As I walked round, I realized that Mary would see the children grow up, she would be at their weddings and I would miss out. In fact I felt severely threatened by all of my female friends and relations! I know they will forgive me now for all these thoughts, but they were real and must be recorded.

Arriving home, even Anthony felt down, and he had been responding with all the positiveness he could muster. The doorbell rang—it was Andrew, the husband of my friend Gillian, acting as postman on her behalf. Gillian is a quiet, thoughtful and sensitive person who possesses a deep faith in God. She had a deep assurance that God would restore my health and had sent me a verse from the book of Proverbs which has become very precious: 'Trust in the Lord with all your heart, and lean not on your own understanding.'

Gillian's letter arrived just when we needed encouragement. I was so thrilled to be reminded that our God knows all our needs, and knows when we need encouragement. Two days later the postman came with a parcel. Inside was a beautiful jumper—also from Gillian.

I christened this my 'love-jumper'. I admit to having a weakness for knitwear and have a cupboard bulging with jumpers. To think that someone thought I might live long enough to warrant having another one was a great boost. That jumper symbolized friendship, love and hope and, whenever I wear it, I thank God for the many ways he has demonstrated his love and care for me, despite my own wavering thoughts and feelings towards him.

Chapter 4
LITTLE REVELATIONS

Like most busy mums, sitting still for half an hour was not
my style. Yet one Tuesday in June after lunch, when
Anthony and Rebecca were napping, I found myself
relaxing in an armchair. Instead of feeling guilty, and
making mental lists of all the things I could be doing, I
found myself opening my mind and heart to God: 'Lord,
help me to make sense out of this situation.' I didn't hear
an audible voice, but into my head poured the words of a
hymn that I hadn't sung for a long time—

> 'Take my life and let it be
> Consecrated, Lord, to Thee.'

It is a hymn in which every part of our being is
dedicated to God's service. When I came to the verse:

> 'Take my voice, and let me sing
> Ever, only for my king,
> Take my lips and they shall be
> Filled with messages from Thee.'

I had to question the Lord, 'How? How can you use
my voice?' Deep within I sensed that he wanted me to
use this period of enforced silence to come quietly to him
and receive more from him. He would teach me and

prepare me for a special task in which I could serve him, but first I had to be led into a new commitment. Peace flooded through me. Hope for a new and exciting future exhilarated me. It was reflected in a letter I wrote to my cousin, Penny, which she photocopied so that, on the 'bad days', I could re-read it:

Dear Penny,
Today I keep crying, but they are not tears of frustration, desolation or hopelessness, they are tears of joy at the way the Lord is moving in our lives. After lunch today, I experienced for the first time the Lord ministering to me. I was sitting quietly, relaxing in the armchair—Anthony was asleep, so was Becca—and I opened my mind to the Lord. He filled it! I am being shown that I need space and time to be restored inwardly, that during that time the hurts and wounds deep down inside are, and will be, dealt with. I was given so clearly the words of a hymn I haven't sung for years, 'Take my life and let it be...' The Lord showed me areas of my life where he has been left on the fringes and as I went through the hymn I could see a new way of living. I asked him—what about 'Take my voice and let me sing... take my lips...'? Could this be physical healing? I believe it may be...eventually. I think the Lord wants me to work with handicapped children, with or without a voice...

Anthony's faith is becoming more vibrant and obvious daily. He strongly believes that I shall be healed even if it is not immediately. The Lord is moving in Claire also—she told me on Sunday that we must all have the peace that passes understanding in our hearts because she has got it in hers! Anthony, Claire and Rebecca have a 'prayer meeting' each night, and yesterday morning, before school, Claire was praying with Rebecca behind the cowsheds. (Sorry about the writing, but I'm excited!)

The prayer support is wonderful—and last night we had a visit from a couple in the village—our age, children at school, who go to Fal. Baptist. They want to come regularly and pray with us.

Today in town was funny. I've become used to not saying more than necessary, but momentarily forgot, and started chatting to a complete stranger about showerproof jackets. (I was getting a cagoule for Anthony.) I was half-way through when I realized that it really only sounded as if I had a bad cold! (It does vary though. When I'm tense it gets worse.)

We saw our family doctor yesterday. He is a Christian and he said to us that he 'has seen strange things happen', that I'm very young to get this—it's usually people in their fifties and sixties.

So, without being unrealistic, we are positive, and for our family the situation is opening up new realms of experience.

Probably you are in tears as well by now!

Love to all,

Cousin Jenny

X

Keep on praying!

A few days later a friend, Mike, arrived. I had known him for years as he belonged to my home church, but I hadn't seen him for a long time. On this and later visits Mike came armed with helpful Christian books, a glowing inner peace and an obvious growing faith—all sources of great encouragement.

On Fridays Anthony goes to bed early in preparation for Saturday's 5.30 a.m. milking, so at 9.30 p.m. that Friday I started reading the book Mike had brought me. It was called *When the Spirit Comes* by Colin Urquhart. At midnight I was still feverishly leafing the pages. I found that as I read more about the transforming power of God's Holy Spirit, a great excitement stirred within me. I felt on the verge of something...a new adventure with God. As a churchgoer from birth, and a committed Christian, I was familiar with references to 'God, the Father, God, the Son, and God, the Holy Spirit' but I had never really considered the role of the Holy Spirit in a Christian's life.

On the following Sunday we attended an open-air service in a local playing-field. It was a well-attended occasion with a band and plenty of warm, June sunshine. It was one verse of a hymn that 'spoke' to me:

'Freedom give to those in bondage,
Lift the burdens caused by sin,
Give new hope, new strength and courage,
Grant release from fears within:
Light for darkness, joy for sorrow;
Love for hatred, peace for strife.
These and countless blessings follow
As the Spirit gives new life.'

I certainly needed release. Physically I longed for my tongue to be released, but I was beginning to understand that spiritual release was equally important, release from the negative feelings of guilt, sorrow and fear.

At this time I was visited by Miriam, one of God's faithful and determined workers. She was so sure of the message she had to bring me: I had to let God deal with my grief. She pointed out to me the words of Jesus, recorded in Luke's Gospel:

'...he has chosen me to bring
    good news to the poor.
He has sent me to proclaim liberty to
    the captives
and recovery of sight to the blind;
to set free the oppressed
and announce the time has come
when the Lord will save his people.

Again it seemed God was telling me about my need to

be released, to be healed in my spirit, to be 'whole' in myself. Was this inner healing the key to enjoying the fullness of life Jesus offered?

During this time of spiritual challenge, we joined people from other churches for a boat trip up the River Fal. I suppose we were a typical group of Cornish Methodists, tucking into our pasties and singing Wesley hymns, huddled in jumpers against the fresh sea air. Among this party were Roderick and Ann. They are related to me in a complicated way so I had met them before, now and again. I felt a little wary of getting involved in conversation: my voice was an embarrassment and I wasn't sure of how my emotions would fare if I embarked on an explanation of my illness. Yet, as our trip progressed, I knew I had to go over and chat with them. It was the first of many occasions when the Lord used me, despite my limitations, to speak to someone. It was as if he took over my unlovely speech, and I found myself telling Ann not only about my illness but also about the strength I was finding as I prayed. I told her my recent realization about the need for inner healing and told her about the book I had read. It was the beginning of a friendship which has led Ann to type the script for this book.

It was much later that I realized just how timely was our conversation that evening. During the previous week Ann had experienced bleak depression, but the Spirit of God was to transform her. I quote from one of her letters:

'Did I tell you that when you first told me of your illness I immediately shouted at my miserable self that this should be me... Then the Lord told me that there was no point in this way of thinking, and to build myself up in positive thoughts for you, and be effective in prayer and action. I can never begin to really express just how much your compassion to me lifted me to a new life in Christ...'

26

If it had been left to me I would have sat dithering and silent on the deck. It was God who used me in my weakness and it was this compassion that touched Ann's heart. It seems that only when we stop relying on our own props, and totally rely on God, can he use us effectively. Without the clutter of self, his love has a chance to shine through. It's expressed very plainly in Mark's Gospel when Jesus is talking about what it means to be his followers:

> '*If anyone wants to come with me, he must forget self, carry his cross, and follow me. For whoever wants to save his own life will lose it; but whoever loses his own life for me and for the gospel will save it.*'

Through illness many of my props were being forced away. To give them up willingly involves an even fiercer battle.

Chapter 5
HOSPITAL VISITS

If you had asked me to list my chief fears in life, the three things I would have said were having to stay in hospital; flying in an aeroplane; and having my ears pierced. All three were to be experienced in the next few months! Our first call to the National Hospital for Neurological Diseases in London coincided with Rebecca's fourth birthday: July 1988. Although the last place I wanted to be on that day was 250 miles away, I couldn't turn down the chance to see Professor Marsden, an expert on MND.

Our appointment was on a Thursday, so we had to travel on the Wednesday—the very day of Rebecca's first afternoon at school. As we turned off the motorway and drove through Windsor, small children were trotting out of school. Guilt and disappointment swamped me. Negative thoughts punched me. I should be greeting Rebecca now as she ran out from school for the first time; I should be there to admire her soggy painting, to take her home and give her orange squash and biscuits...this wretched disease was robbing my children of the Mum they deserved.

We stayed with friends in Wimbledon. Pam and I had been neighbours at the age of four and had had adjoining bedrooms in semi-detached houses. At night we would tap signals on the wall and even made plans to cut a hole so we could climb to and fro. Together we weathered tots' tantrums and teenage traumas so, although we'd never visited them in Wimbledon before, it immediately seemed like home. Their two-year-old daughter, Sheridan, was a delightful diversion from hospital thoughts with her non-stop repertoire of songs and questions.

Just after nine on Thursday morning we were sitting in Queens Square just outside the hospital. It was a pretty garden and people were still hurrying to work. There everything seemed so natural and normal that I felt reluctant to leave it for the unknown corridors of the brick building behind.

A young doctor saw me first and, after a barrage of questions, I was subjected to rigorous physical tests; it seemed to involve pitting my strength against that of the doctor as he pushed and pulled my limbs. At times I felt as if I was auditioning for a wrestling contest! All the time, though, a Bible verse kept running through my head. Isaiah said:

> 'But those who trust in the Lord for help
> will find their strength renewed.
> They will rise on wings like eagles;
> they will run and not get weary;
> they will walk and not grow weak.'

At last we were called into Professor Marsden's large consulting room. He quietly confirmed the diagnosis of MND but, in order to make absolutely sure, wanted me to return in a few weeks as an in-patient to undergo further tests. Panic rose. I hoped that perhaps the world would end before my appointment came through!

We sat in the Square again. It was warm and sunny, and hospital staff were picnicking on the grass. It was time to take a deep breath—what now? We had each hoped that it wasn't MND and that we could have been sent away with a magic formula to bring back my voice. I told Anthony about that insistent verse from Isaiah.

There was no cure for MND but in those words was our key to survival. It was time to set off again, our hands tightly gripped in God's hands, trusting him for strength and direction.

We decided to have some lunch and then head for the London Healing Mission in Notting Hill. We had been told about it by a friend. I had imagined it would be a hall built in red brick, but in fact it was a huge house in a residential area. As the door opened a savoury dinner-time smell wafted out, and we were directed to the basement where a healing service was taking place. It had almost finished and people were quietly walking to the front of the little chapel where members of 'the team' were talking and praying with them. What immediately struck me was the calm, warm atmosphere—the peace of God was almost tangible. We were ushered forward and met Yvonne. It was the first time for both of us that we had experienced such searching and powerful prayer. Here was someone totally open to God and 'tuned in' to him. We felt shaken when she prayed about areas of hurt in my life that she obviously couldn't have known about—it was like a knife probing deep within. Also, when she prayed, she prayed with authority, rebuking the disease in the name of Jesus, so that we felt physically shaken by the words. It was a new insight into the work of the Holy Spirit: this was God's Holy Spirit moving in 'Acts of the Apostles' style—no longer relegated to a nebulous third part of the Trinity.

As Anthony and I left the Mission we felt both drained and filled. We were physically, mentally and emotionally tired after all the morning's events, and yet that afternoon God had touched our lives, demonstrated his power and given us a special unexplainable peace and hope.

Through our friends God continued to meet our needs and even give us treats. While we were away we heard that one friend had given us an answering machine so I wouldn't have to worry about making myself under-stood on the phone. Then along came Pam with the tickets for *Phantom of the Opera*, a London show fully booked for months ahead! It was a marvellous evening: we were able to sit totally engrossed in the story and marvel at the spectacular set while the music swept over us. For two-and-a-half hours we forgot about hospital appointments and missed birthdays. It was a wonderful present from God.

Home-coming was not easy. I was really looking forward to seeing the children and thought they would be equally pleased to see us. Instead it took two or three days for them to settle down. They were fractious, distant. It seemed as if they were punishing us for leaving them, despite the good time they had had with their grandparents. Again guilt and fear set in. Was I making their lives insecure? What if they didn't love me any more?

One of the first messages to be left on our answering machine was from the London Hospital. They had reserved a bed for me for Monday 1 August, much earlier than we had expected. We had four days to make arrangements. My cousin Penny and her family, who were due to arrive for a week's holiday, promptly offered to take charge of the house and children while I was away. This was a great relief. The children thought Aunty Penny 'was funny' so I knew they would be happy. Anthony was in the midst of the corn harvest, making it impossible for him to leave the farm, so his mother offered to accompany me up on the train. She was always quick to give practical help when a need arose. It was agreed that Anthony would join me as soon as he could.

For four days at the hospital I was questioned and prodded by numerous doctors, most of whom were approachable and understanding. There was just one who used to mutter medical phrases that I only half understood and which sent me into hyper-ventilation! Also, of course, there were the tests: one scan involved my whole body being shuttled into a narrow tunnel, with my head tightly encased in an even smaller space while the Beatles yelled in my ears, 'Help, I need somebody!' presumably to allay any feelings of claustrophobia. I spent twenty minutes entombed with the Liverpool lads. The second test was good preparation for acu4puncture, should I desire it. Needles were stuck into different places in my arms and legs and little electric currents passed through them—not very pleasant. The final test was more relaxing: I had to recline in a semi-dark room while my limbs were wired up to a machine that took readings of muscle movements. I may have looked like an exhibit from the Dr Who museum, but I felt quite relaxed!

The worst aspect of the four days was that I couldn't escape and have a good cry. Motor Neurone Disease makes it difficult to control emotions and I felt extremely embarrassed about bursting into tears with sick people all around me. I wanted to explain to them that I couldn't help it, that I knew they were ill too. It was humiliating.

Being a long way from home without Anthony I could so easily have been lonely, but the stream of cards, flowers and visitors flowing to my corner of the ward were a source of amazement to everyone and another sign of God's provision. Lynn wrote so often that I knew every move and meal for a week—in fact her letters continued to be forwarded after I had returned home! In four days I had fourteen visitors and three deliveries of flowers.

The outstanding memories of that week were the other women in my part of the ward. Liz was a young West Indian girl who had gone into a coma when a school teacher failed to recognize the seriousness of an asthma attack. She was partially paralyzed and very bitter. For her the future lay in getting revenge.

Next to me lay Edith—able only to smile. She had been like that for twelve years. I watched as staff did everything for her, sometimes even singing her nursery rhymes. I felt indignant for her indignity. Her husband came one day: you could sense his genuine love for her; she was still his Edith, the one he had loved and married. No others came. After twelve years there were no cards or letters. No flowers for Edith.

Then there was Peggy. She was about sixty, a single lady who lived alone. She had great difficulty walking and was undergoing tests. They gave her no hope of improvement and on the day she was due to leave she was extremely depressed and suicidal. She could find no hope in the future: she didn't know how she was going to cope, and was afraid of being lonely. 'I'd be better out of it,' she told me.

My heart ached for Peggy and I wanted to tell her that Jesus cared about how she felt, that he had died to take away all her grief and fear, that each day he would give her special peace and strength if she would ask. I locked myself into the bathroom and prayed, 'Lord, I can't speak to Peggy. Show me how to give her your love.' Soon I was back on my bed writing to her. The words flowed. I believe it was God's special message for Peggy. Just before she left I gave her the letter to open when she got home. It was the start of a beautiful pen-friendship. A few weeks later she wrote telling me how that letter had helped her and how, far from being lonely, friends were rallying round. Recently she wrote to say she had been diagnosed as having Multiple Sclerosis but she continued: 'I just say my prayers and ask for help to see me through each day.'

Anthony had arrived on the Thursday and before we left one of the senior doctors spoke to us. Yes, I had Motor Neurone Disease but there were certain aspects that didn't follow the normal pattern: I was younger than most sufferers; my voice had degenerated quickly and there was no sign of muscle wasting elsewhere. Nothing had been gained or lost and it was with a great sense of freedom that we walked down to Covent Garden, browsing in the shops and taking refreshment in the noisy, open-air cafe. It was such a relief to be an anonymous visitor in the cosmopolitan city crowd: for an hour I could have been anyone instead of Jenny Richards who had been declared victim of MND by three different experts.

When we arrived home Penny stayed on for a few days. I thought it would be my chance to give her a holiday. She could sit down while I did all the cooking and tidying. But when I got home I felt like a rag and was equally useless. I ended up lying pathetically in bed while she packed a picnic and again took responsibility for the tribe! It was in this state, though, that I received what I called my first 'poem of the Spirit'. The words flowed into my mind...

> 'I am cradled in a cocoon of my Creator's
>   healing love.
> My Spirit is released—it soars and sings.
> Silently, soothingly muscles are massaged—
> They relax and gain strength.
>
> Suddenly the cocoon bursts open—
> Body and Spirit sing and dance before the Lord—
> Hallelujah! Thank you, Jesus!'

In my weakness, God had inspired me. His words had encouraged me and, in time, were to strengthen others.

Chapter 6
PRAYERS FOR HEALING

'There are times when prayer is the only gift we can give one another,' said the card in my hand. We had been showered by gifts of prayer from many different people. The faithfulness of people's praying continually touched us and has been a source of immense hope and strength. It is very moving and humbling when people who only know me by name assure us of daily prayer, and when prayer groups in London and Leeds and even Australia and New Zealand tell us of their prayers for us each week at their meetings.

When afflicted by a disease labelled 'terminal' it is easy to feel a frantic desperation to find a cure: running against the clock to beat the disease. Yet right from the start I didn't want the quality of our family life to become overtaken by endless ventures into alternative medicines, and I prayed also that God would guide us and give us discernment as we sought prayers for healing. It has been wonderful to see how he has provided the right people to pray with us in moments of special need.

Kea Church, about three miles away from our home, regularly set time aside during their services for healing prayer. One Sunday evening, my friend Gillian and I decided to go along and it was there that I met Bob Redrup, the vicar, and Mary Richards, the ordained deacon. As soon as Mary saw me she said, 'Have you had a shock?' The question toppled my emotional poise. I burst into tears and with Gillian's help explained about Dad's sudden death at Christmas. Normally I would have felt embarrassed about crying in front of strangers, but the love in their words and on their faces assured me that we were family—God's family. As they laid hands on me and prayed, a warmth and peace again flowed through me. They had recognized my need for inner healing and invited me to another special healing service on a following Sunday morning.

The healing service coincided with Penny's stay, so she went with me. This time Bob questioned me about the occult—had I or any of my family been involved? No they hadn't. Then Penny remembered something that had happened to me at the end of my probationary year of teaching before I returned to Cornwall to teach. It was at a very rough comprehensive school in Essex and in one of my third-year classes were three rather unpleasant girls. At the end of my last lesson with them they encircled me and chanted 'We hope you have a horrible life.' It upset me, but I didn't think that I had let it really disturb my thinking about the future. Bob felt it was right to break any powers this curse had over me and prayed with power and authority in the name of Jesus.

Mary Richards was due to leave Kea Church to take up a new post in Bristol very soon, but before she went she generously gave her time for three prayer sessions with me. They were painful, for we had to uproot those deep-seated hurts inside and let Jesus pour in the healing balm of his love. Several areas of hurt emerged.

The first was the death of my maternal grandfather—'Ga-Ga' as I called him. One January afternoon when I was four I was sent up to the vegetable patch to call Ga-Ga for tea. I followed him to the shed door while he put his tools away. As he propped up the fork against the wall, he seemed to lean on it and then crumple to the floor. I remember running down the path screaming. The next thing I was gathered into someone's arms, whisked out of the back gate and deposited with a neighbour. It is so vivid. Mary prayed through the experience, allaying any anxiety or guilt I might have felt. As she prayed she kept reminding me that Jesus had been there holding that little girl's hand, and lovingly receiving Ga-Ga into his eternal Kingdom.

The next area we dealt with was my Dad's death, because although almost thirty years after Ga-Ga's, the manner of death was similar. As I handed Dad an early morning cup of tea, he sat up and then fell backwards across the bed. I was caught between alerting help and wanting to do something for Dad. I raced for the bedroom, phoned for the doctor and then for Anthony. Then I tried to move Dad into a better position, desperately rubbing his back and praying, 'Don't let him die!' Anthony was home within minutes and could immediately see that Dad was past reviving. When the doctor came he assured me that there was nothing I could have done. Yet I was beset with guilt: maybe I should have moved him before dashing for the phone. Should I have noticed that he was ill weeks earlier? Should I have done more housework, cooking, shopping for him? The guilt was increased when I attended 'Save a Life' courses in order to teach swimming. Every time we worked on the dummy, learning mouth to mouth resuscitation, I thought that maybe if I'd known all this at Christmas, I could have saved Dad. Again, Mary prayed through these events with me, assuring me of God's presence with me and my Dad. Gradually the painful grief and the guilt were taken away. I was able to feel peaceful about my role in the events, and start enjoying the good memories of my Dad.

In a similar way Mary helped me to let God deal with the deep-seated grief and hurt over Mum's death. The sense of loss was still sharp: I didn't just miss her for myself—I missed her for my children. She loved children and would have derived great delight from Claire and Rebecca. She was a great story-teller, and had a keen sense of fun. I so wished that the children could have known her. Guilt again reared its head. It seemed to me that she had worked so hard to see me through school and that I didn't have the chance to repay her. I would have loved to entertain her in our home and give her some treats for a change. It took many months of talking, crying and praying before the 'Mum' hurt subsided and still the Lord is dealing with it.

These experiences of inner healing prompted another poem:

Tangles

This morning I combed Claire's hair,
The comb bit into the tangled ends.
Claire protested, hating the tugging and hurting,
Impatient to get away.

Lord, I am hurting as the tangles of my life are pulled
    apart.
I too struggle and am impatient to be released.

Claire's hair is smooth and beautiful,
She smiles at her reflection.
Lord, when my untangling is complete,
Let me smile at your reflection
In the mirror of my life.

At the end of August we were summoned to our local specialist again. We knew how depressing the visit could be and prayed that God would protect us. As we entered the doctor's room he didn't greet us in any way: instead he studied the reports from London and said, 'This is grim, very grim indeed.' The atmosphere of gloom continued as he spelled out how I would deteriorate: when I couldn't speak at all, I could write; when I couldn't write—there'd be a problem; when I couldn't eat ordinary food, I could liquidize everything. The outcome was inevitable: there was no room for miracles.

I believe that, if I hadn't had the strength and peace of God and the support of Christian family and friends, I would have been suicidal. Instead, as the consultation progressed, Anthony and I had to stifle laughter: we didn't believe that we had to accept this negative outlook. God was giving us victory—in and over our situation—and, on this occasion, it was expressed in our laughter.

Soon after, some friends invited me to attend a healing meeting at the Elim Church in Falmouth. It was part of a week of mission led by special people. The main speaker was renowned for his spiritual insight and his gift of prophecy—an ability given by God to speak out God's words in a particular situation—so when he invited people to come up on the platform for healing, I was the first there. I handed him a bit of paper that explained my predicament. After laying hands on me and praying for healing he announced to the congregation that I would regain my voice in a few days, and that I would be used to bring the gospel to people from different countries, and that I was not to be anxious about money. I do not regret attending the meeting but I am still mystified by most of the prophecy. My voice didn't return within a few days and I haven't yet had the opportunity to reach people from other countries— unless this book is published in different languages! However, the Lord has looked after us financially. Whereas, on paper, having no income from my job meant that outgoings exceeded incomings, our needs have been met and on many occasions we have found ourselves on the receiving end of terrific generosity. A third of the prophecy had been fulfilled. Dare I hope for the rest?

Chapter 7
ONLY THE BEST

At the end of the summer, courtesy of the Health Service, I gained a great new friend—'my machine'. It is three hundred pounds' worth of slim-line technology designed by a disabled person who is unable to speak. Officially called a lightwriter, it has a small typing keyboard and two little screens. As I type in my words, The person sitting opposite and I can read what I'm 'saying'. This re-opened my world of conversation: it meant that I could chat to other mums at the school gate; I could say what I really wanted to say to my friends instead of choosing the shortest, easiest words; I could ask for things in shops without preparing endless written notes.

I was surprised and delighted by people's reactions. They weren't at all embarrassed: even strangers who asked the way read the words and went off in the right direction. In shops I did find that, although the assistants were fascinated, they assumed I was deaf and answered me with exaggerated mouth movements and wild gesticulation. I solved this by showing a little card which said: 'I cannot speak, but I can hear.' My machine has become an object of affection, attracting various names: Rebecca calls it 'Mummy's dooter'; Claire calls it a 'beeper' and Lynn refers to it as my 'humdinger'.

As my voice deteriorated, Claire learnt to understand my funny sounds: she would watch me carefully and often translated for her friends and for Rebecca. At the age of six she was displaying immense sensitivity. For Rebecca at just four, it was more difficult: she couldn't concentrate like Claire, and attempts at conversation often ended with us both in tears of frustration.

As a teacher I knew the importance of reading in developing language skills and felt very guilty for no longer being able to read to the children. In Claire's pre-school days we had enjoyed so many books together. As the time approached for the school term to begin I worried about the effect my lack of voice would have on Becca's development. Would I be the cause of some kind of backwardness? I needn't have worried. She relished everything about school and was soon eager to show me that even if I couldn't read to her, she could tell me what lots of different words were! In my situation I have had to learn to entrust my children into God's care, to trust him to provide the things I cannot. I have to continually remind myself of another verse from Isaiah:

> 'I will pour out my power on your children
> and my blessings on your descendants.
> They will thrive like well-watered grass,
> like willows by streams of running water.'

At six o'clock one October morning, armed with my machine and my intense feelings of guilt and anxiety over the children, Gillian and I set off on the train for a day trip to London where we had an appointment to see the Reverend Andy Arbuthnot at the London Healing Mission. Since that first visit in July, I had written to Andy, usually when feeling low, asking him questions which he has probably encountered innumerable times before. Yet I always received a prompt reply; always he wrote as to a special friend showing genuine compassion, always the love of Christ flowed through his words, encouraging, up-lifting and sometimes challenging me.

Anthony clearly remembers the first communication I had with Andy. It was a Wednesday—Truro Market Day. When Anthony left me I was rather down and he felt distressed that he couldn't cheer me up. The phone rang. It was Andy, who had felt compelled to ring. It didn't matter that I could say almost nothing; he brought the love of Jesus to me that afternoon. As he prayed over the phone, I felt the warmth of Jesus' presence and knew that he did care for me. At my worst moments I might feel abandoned by God, but in fact he held me in his arms—he had something special in store for me. When Anthony returned, he saw a different person!

Consultations at the Mission usually last one hour, but, considering the distance we had travelled, ours was a generous two hours. I did a lot of tapping on my machine, and the box of tissues strategically positioned by my chair was also well used. Andy soon recognized the deep grief I felt about the children and counselled me in letting them go—to God. I remember standing with Andy and Gillian either side of me, my arms outstretched, and being 'shown' Jesus standing in front of me. His arms were outstretched to receive and take away my pain, to receive and take care of my children, to give me his peace and his love.

Two things Andy said to me stayed in my mind: the first was 'Jesus and Jenny will win.' Whenever I feel deserted and alone in my illness I try to recall this partnership. Jesus is there with me in the darkness, knowing totally the intense hurt, but leading me to victory. He knows every step and pitfall on the way of the cross, but he also invites me to experience resurrection power—the power that refuses to be crushed by the physical limitations of suffering, the power that looks forward with certainty to eventual wholeness of body, mind and spirit. For me it is well-expressed in the final verse of a hymn:

Then shall I see, and hear, and know
All I desired or wished below;
And every power find sweet employ
In that eternal world of joy!

That's something to look forward to!

The other thing Andy said was, 'Jesus doesn't want you to have second best.' This has provoked many questions from me to God: 'If you only want what's best, Lord, then why am I like this? Why aren't I healed? Surely at my best I could be preaching, teaching, doing so many things for you?' Then comes the uncomfortable feeling that maybe this is his best for me. 'Is this how you can use me best, Lord? Really? Well, if so, can it just be for a few months, or a year? After that, would you make me fully fit again? Yes, I'm happy to be used in this way for a *short* time...'

Andy lent me a tape by a woman called Joni. She had been paralyzed in an accident and, despite having many assurances from friends that she would be healed, and having faith in herself, she remained wheelchair bound. Yet God uses her now in a remarkable way. She preaches from her wheelchair world-wide and those who see her say that her disabilities fade into the background, as the light of Jesus shines from her face.

Joni is living out God's best for her. Above all she gladly accepts his plan for her life. Her testimony made me think, 'Who am I to dictate to God what is best for me?' I had to be willing for him to use me with no voice—for as long as he chose.

Two days after this visit to the mission, I was faced with a dilemma. We had been invited to Anthony's cousin's wedding. The service was to be held in Camborne Wesley Church—the place where we had married and where my father's funeral had taken place nine months before. I also knew that I would be meeting some friends that I hadn't seen since before my illness.

Panic set in. I didn't think I could cope with the service. What if I started to cry and made a fool of myself? Yet I really wanted to take part in the celebration of this lovely Christian marriage. If I didn't go I would be settling for second best, wouldn't I? I would be denying Jesus' partnership. At this point, a marvellous thing happened—Anthony and I prayed together for the first time. It seemed the most natural thing to do. I shall never forget sitting on the bed with Anthony's arm around me, as he claimed God's strength for the hours ahead. It was the start of a new dimension to our marriage.

I think God must have a sense of humour, for when Anthony stood up, there, on the bed, was my new cream hat, rather buckled and bent under his weight! It certainly made us laugh.

We sat at the back of the church and I did have a little weep initially. During the hymns and taking of vows I held my hymn-sheet over my trembling lips, but I know that Jesus was beside me in the pew, giving me his victory. At the end of the reception I could honestly say I had had a good time. I had experienced Jesus' best for me that day.

On the following day I attended the evening service at our chapel in Frogpool. One of our ministers was preaching and, although I can't remember now what he actually said, as the service continued I had a growing conviction that I had to start preaching again. This conviction wouldn't go away. As the week progressed it kept nagging me. But how could I preach with no voice? Then a picture formed in my mind. I was preparing the service, I was standing in the pulpit, but there was someone else doing the speaking. It was Anthony! Now Anthony hated public speaking, his knees knocked at the thought of reading a lesson at Christmas. Yet this picture was as insistent as the call to preach and I knew I had to tell Anthony. God had obviously been preparing him, because, instead of reacting in shocked horror, he smiled and said if that was what God wanted, then who was he to argue. I immediately wrote to our minister, explaining this call to preach. He quickly acknowledged the letter, but decided to wait until the New Year before making definite arrangements. He wanted us both to be sure of our calling.

At the end of October we had another appointment with our specialist at Truro. What a contrast to our previous visit! This time he accepted that there was no further deterioration and for the first time expressed a hope that the disease might have arrested—a very rare phenomenon! A little optimism crept into his voice: if things were the same in January, he wouldn't need to see me again.

If it really had arrested, then we knew it was because God had intervened, and if God could arrest a disease, he could also rebuild destroyed neurons and wasted muscles. We rejoiced! It was on this theme of rebuilding and transformation that I wrote another poem:

The Pool

A disabled girl came to the pool today,
She limped awkwardly down the steps,
One arm dangling uselessly by her side.
Then she lunged forward,
Abandoning herself to the water...
I watched as its buoyancy transformed her,
She moved freely, gracefully
And happiness shone in her eyes.

Father, I limp towards you,
Weak and exhausted from pain, weeping and fear,
Silent.
Immerse me in your love,
For it is only your love that can hold me up.
Let your love transform me.
I want to live freely and strongly for you,

I want to shout out your words,
And feel the thrill of singing your praises.
I want others to see the ripple of your laughter
in my eyes,
As you look lovingly upon your re-creation,
And rejoice.

Chapter 8
CHRISTMAS 1988

From August onwards I had felt pangs of dread every time I thought about Christmas. It would be the first Christmas without Dad and indeed it would mark the anniversary of his death. It also marked the end of one year of my illness and, according to the specialist's prognosis, could easily be my last. I felt no desire for the usual festivities, yet I wanted it to be special for us as a family. Although I hadn't mentioned this to anyone, it was Anthony's mother who displayed sensitivity and selflessness when she suggested that we went away for Christmas. She understood how difficult it would be for me, and, although their own Christmas would be quieter, thought it was an ideal solution.

Apart from trips to Paris as children, Anthony and I had not been abroad. Neither of us had ever flown, so it was quite an adventure when, on 22 December, we set off on a four-hour flight to Lanzarote. Such was the seating that I had to sit next to two strangers, and I was a bit concerned about conversation. But God had the seating in hand, for, as soon as I sat down and put my machine on my lap, the lady next to me recognized it. She taught children who used these lightwriters and was quite at ease talking and 'listening' to me. She and her husband were well-travelled and, as the plane took off and my stomach took a while to catch up with the rest of me, they gave me confidence for the hours in the air!

We landed in the late afternoon heat and from then on it was like a summer holiday instead of Christmas, apart from a miniature Christmas cake we had been given and the Germans in the resort singing 'Silent Night'. It was something so very different from anything we had done before and I believe God used the time to build us up in different ways.

It increased Anthony's confidence. After leaving school, he had lived and worked at home on the farm, attending a local college part-time, so that he never had to fend for himself. Even on our family holidays I usually and gladly did the arranging and enquiries. Anthony felt more comfortable in a supporting role. Here in Lanzarote, where we knew no one, he had total responsibility for two young children and a wife who couldn't speak, and might on occasions choke. He was great. He took control of the shopping and of the cooking. His fried eggs and fritters became a family favourite. He 'covered' for my lack of voice by chatting to other tourists in the queue for the excursion coaches which arrived according to whim rather than timetable. He swotted up on useful Spanish sayings and manfully used them. (There was just one lapse when, on arrival at our complex, he said 'Merci' to the Spanish mini-bus driver.)

For two weeks we had time together as a family unit— a valuable experience for anyone. Of course the children preferred to play in the pool with new-found friends most of the time, but we still went on excursions, read books, played games and listened to tapes together. Months later Rebecca will suddenly recall a holiday memory—usually something to do with the camel ride. It meant that Anthony and I had a lot of time to talk and pray. The events of the previous Christmas were by no means blotted out by the sun and Anthony lovingly and patiently encouraged me to talk about it. As I relived the events I believe the shock of Dad's death went at last. We also talked more about Mum; Anthony encouraged me to talk about her to the children, recalling the happy, funny things.

I was also able to tell Anthony about my growing fears for him. I felt such a burden. What if the worry about me affected his health? I just needed assurances that he was all right, and that if ever he felt ill he would see a doctor. Condemnation is a tool much-used by God's enemies. Tempting us to condemn ourselves keeps us down. I have been very prone to this, blaming myself for adversely affecting the lives of those I love. I ought to have a verse from the New Testament, from Paul's letter to the Romans, written on the back of my hand:

'There is no condemnation now for those who live in union with Christ Jesus.'

If God doesn't condemn me, who am I to condemn myself?

Praying together was a relatively new experience and praying aloud was totally new to Anthony. Yet God continually used Anthony to enrich my prayer life. At times when I have been too upset or tired or puzzled to be able to formulate prayers, the Spirit of God has prompted Anthony to pray the things deep in my heart. In these prayer times God seems to bind us even tighter together and to himself with his love.

In almost ten years of marriage, I had longed to pray together but had been reticent in suggesting it. Now I longed to partake more vocally. Anthony always encouraged me to pray aloud: he said it didn't matter that he didn't understand—God would—but I hated the ugly voice struggling to say things. I preferred to add my own prayers silently. Once or twice I used my machine to tap out prayers, but nothing seemed to compensate for a voice with which to pray aloud. How could my praying encourage Anthony if he couldn't hear me? I had to trust the Holy Spirit to be our communicator.

Above all, we were able to have a good time. As I flick through the photograph album, all kinds of memories flood through my mind: the fierce wind that blew orange Sahara dust into our hair and clothes; the eerie and fantastic sights in the volcanic park; the ungracious camel ride; the sun on the Green Lagoon; the fields of cacti and the fate of the cochineal beetle; farmers working the arid land with donkeys and camels; the pink glow of a disused salt mine; Claire sitting still and serious while a street artist charcoaled her portrait; Anthony diving into the pool to rescue Rebecca's doll's shoes!

For me the outstanding memory is something that happened when we visited some volcanic caves in the north of the island. Our guide brought us to the edge of what appeared to be a deep precipice: he asked us to listen as he threw down a pebble. We expected to hear the sounds as it fell down over the rocks: instead it went 'plop' and landed in a shallow pool of water. The precipice hadn't existed: it was merely a reflection in the water of the craggy cave roof. As we walked out of the caves, I knew God was telling me something. It came in the form of another poem:

In the Caves

Our guide led us through the eerie, volcanic caves
Deep underground.
Suddenly his arm shot out—
'Stand well back!' he shouted.
We stood at the edge of an endless abyss of sharp, dark rocks.
Parents grabbed their children,
A protective husband pulled back his wife.
The guide held up a pebble.
'Listen,' he whispered and threw it down into the depths...

Plop! went the pebble as a shallow pool of water
    shimmered before us.
No danger here—merely a reflection of the cave's
    roof.

There are times in our lives, Lord,
When we stand in front of seemingly unfathomable
    depths,
Insoluble problems, interminable pain, endless
    darkness.
Then you drop your love into our lives,
It shimmers and spreads through our whole being,
Until the fears, the hurts, the darkness
that seemed so huge and real,
Are no longer there.
Instead there is light and peace and radiating joy.
You are our loving Father
It is you who is real
And we are safe—in your love.

It was during our holiday that we started to doubt
that the disease had arrested. I had two falls, got bad
cramp in my legs at night, and my left foot felt awkward
as I walked. We tried to think up other reasons for these
things: perhaps I had walked further than usual, perhaps
I was slightly dehydrated, but inside we both knew that
this was a sign of leg muscle wasting.

Within a few days of being home we had our appointment with the specialist. He thoroughly examined my
legs and arms and could detect no sign of deterioration.
To him it appeared that the disease had arrested and he
dismissed us without further appointments. I tried to be
relieved, and kept telling people what the specialist had
said, hoping it was true, but couldn't ignore what was
happening to me. It was increasingly difficult to walk.
The disease was surely on the march again. I needed all
the assurance expressed in my poem. God had to be
more real to me than this intrusive disease.

Chapter 9
CANDLES IN THE DARKNESS

Between February and July 1989 I lived a physical nightmare. Indeed there were times when I couldn't believe that something so dreadful was happening to me. My ability to walk gradually deteriorated. First it meant that I just walked awkwardly, then slowly, soon even the gentlest incline was a problem and I found myself needing an arm to cling on to. I was given a tripod which steadied me a little and meant that I didn't always need an arm, but much independence had vanished. I could no longer do my shopping alone and even walking down the path to the car took five minutes and was a mammoth expedition.

As my legs weakened, so did my arms. My left hand gradually curled up and became useless; I could no longer manipulate a knife and fork, and I had to use just a fork in my right hand. Eventually I didn't have enough strength to lever myself out of the bath or out of a chair. Everyday activities became mountains of difficulty: getting out of bed, dressing, undressing, picking up the pile of washing, hanging out clothes, changing beds, lifting a kettle full of water. Each day something ordinary would become a hurdle.

In May my swallowing became further affected and more foods were crossed off my list. Bread and cake crumbs stuck in my throat and made me choke; cereals had the same effect. I was limited to foods that could be mixed in with mashed potato, or desserts such as mild yoghurts that would slide down easily. Eating even these things took immense concentration and if we were invited to friends for dinner I would eat before or after so I could enjoy their company. They were very understanding.

Not being able to communicate properly with Anthony and the children had been bad enough, but now my ability to look after their physical needs was diminishing, I felt devastated. People sing and talk glibly about broken hearts. This year there have been many occasions when it has felt as if my heart were literally breaking, so painful was the hurt inside. I grieved for the person I used to be, for my lost faculties; I grieved for the wife Anthony had lost, for the Mum Claire and Rebecca had lost, for the friend my friends had lost.

There were times when I wished that I didn't believe in a God who could heal people. It would have been easier. But believing that he could heal, I was then wracked with the question, 'Why not me?' Perhaps there was a reason why he wouldn't heal me. One preacher declared, 'There are no wheelchairs on faith's highway.' So, perhaps it was all my fault—I didn't have enough faith. There were so many questions that whirled around my mind. Any human friend or even acquaintance would make me well in a second if they were able, so why couldn't a loving, heavenly Father be equally compassionate?

Why had the people with the negative outlook on my illness proved to be right? Why hadn't those who believed in and prophesied my healing been right? I tried to remind myself of the truth I thought I had grasped in October—God's best for my life might not be what I considered best for me. But, Lord, how can your best deprive a husband of his wife and children of their mother? How can your best bring so much hurt and heartache? So many questions tangled in my mind. I was walking in 'death's dark vale'. Shepherd, are you really there?

He was. In the physical, mental and often spiritual darkness of these months, there were candles of blessing and encouragement.

In January a family from Australia joined our church—Les and Jackie and their children. They had a faith that sparkled and one evening we invited them to our home. It was great to hear them talk about how God had guided their lives. That evening we prayed together, and for me the Lord answered a ten-year-old prayer— Anthony publicly committed his life to Jesus. I truly felt that my illness had been worthwhile if it had led Anthony to this point of dedication.

The last weekend in February we were bathed in blessing.

On the Friday evening we attended a 'renewal' meeting at St Austell where the speaker preached on 'No Condemnation?' Towards the end of the meeting he encouraged us to minister to each other by placing our hands on the head of the person sitting with us. Anthony placed his hands on my head and started to pray quietly. He experienced the Spirit of God in a completely new way. He said he felt his body tingle and he couldn't stop his arms shaking. He said it was as if the illness was leaving me. He came away from the meeting having had an insight into the Holy Spirit at work and he was thirsty for more. He was also convinced that the root of the illness had left me, that I was healed.

On Saturday I had booked to attend a Day Seminar which was being held nearby. It was on healing and was being led by Andy and Audrey Arbuthnot from the Healing Mission. I was really looking forward to seeing Andy again, and meeting Audrey. My friend Lynn and I attended all day and Anthony joined us for the last two sessions. The last session involved a time of quiet prayer in which the Spirit of God directed the ministry. As we stood there with arms outstretched again Anthony felt led to lay his hands on me. Again he experienced a tremendous in-filling of the Holy Spirit: he was shaking and again his arms tingled. After a time of weeping, I sat still and felt very peaceful. A person behind had put a hand on my shoulder. As people all around were prayed for, a beautiful picture formed in my mind. I saw Jesus holding a huge white box that had been tied with a festive ribbon. The lid was opening and inside I could see a new voice and feet that were swift. They were for me.

Andy then invited anyone who would like to ask for the gift of tongues—one of the gifts of the Holy Spirit— to go into the next room. About ten people moved forward, including Anthony and me. By the middle of that following week my Anthony, man of few words who doesn't go in for fancy expressions, was praying in a beautiful new language that the Holy Spirit had inspired. The gift was so right for him at that time. It has helped him when he hasn't known what or how to pray. It has encouraged me also. God had given Anthony something I could actually hear.

It was after supper that we were eventually able to speak to Andy. He prayed with us and said that he saw a tremendous light in me. Audrey told me that when she had seen me in that earlier time of ministry she had sensed an illness leaving me. I told Andy that I couldn't understand why the illness seemed to have arrested and then progressed again. A thought struck him: had we ever rebuked the original diagnosis and prognosis? In the name of Jesus he broke any hold that 'death sentence' had over me. He also encouraged Anthony to continue laying hands on me: the gift of communicating God's healing love was not reserved for ministers and evangelists.

That weekend we both felt a sense of excitement. We

felt that God was leading us into a new dimension of service and that he would use our varying gifts as we worked together for him. Had Anthony been given the gift of healing?

Anthony had certainly been given boldness. On Easter Sunday morning he did something which six months before he couldn't have imagined—he addressed the children in church. His father was supposed to be preaching, but had been suffering from a bad cold. The day before the service I felt compelled to offer to write the children's address if Anthony would read it. He didn't read it; he told it. He amazed himself and everybody; it was as if it was something he did every week. Such is the power of the Spirit of God. As he told the story, I worked a hand puppet, and held up other visual aids. I had really missed my contact with the Sunday School. It was so good to be able to communicate with them again.

At about the same time our minister was making arrangements for Anthony and me to take services in our Methodist Circuit. Before we could go 'solo'—or 'duet'—we had to be accompanied by an accredited local preacher and I had to enrol on a preacher's examination course which would take two years to complete. This was certainly an act of faith! We were assigned to Celia Philips who accepted her role with enthusiasm and humility. As we prepared and partook in services together we all felt as if we were learning from and giving to each other. I found it more difficult than I had anticipated being the silent and now stumbling partner. I felt rather embarrassed limping into a pew, and then not audibly participating in hymns. Would people who didn't know my situation think I was strange? Such vanity was distracting from my call to preach. God graciously reassured me each time with a person's warm handshake or a word of appreciation and welcome.

In April, John (another of Anthony's many cousins)

and his wife Paula returned from a year in New Zealand where they had been involved in some work with Youth With A Mission—an organization quite unlike the traditional idea of 'missionary' work. At a time when our spirits were flagging they brought a freshness to our situation, and, despite all the people they had to visit, were generous in the time they spent with us.

One Sunday evening they called to find both Anthony and me rather low. Anthony was exhausted after two weeks of silage making, and for the first time in eighteen months had given up any hope of my recovery. We both felt we were failing the children: I, because I couldn't communicate with them adequately; Anthony, because he felt he was taking out his tiredness and frustration on them. We were both too dispirited even to pray. Yet out of this trough came a time of prayer that revived us, and brought Paula a new experience of the Holy Spirit's work. As in all our prayer times, there were times of silence, of listening to God, as well as talking to him, praying and asking, and praising him. As Paula prayed, she felt God was pointing out an insecurity in my life in recent years. As we talked and prayed we saw how the Lord was pin-pointing my sense of insecurity about having no mum to turn to. I had been able to talk about anything to my mum and there had been so many times when I had yearned to turn to her for a word of advice or a just a chat. When friends had their mums to stay after new babies were born, or when they went on shopping expeditions together, or just stayed at home having fun with the children, I used to ache for that relationship.

Having talked about this, we continued praying. Paula then spoke out very loudly and with great authority. She told me how wanted and special I had been to my parents, and how God now wanted to be a mother and father to me. If I turned to him, he would make up to me all that I missed in my earthly parents. Paula said later that never before had she received and delivered a message from God in that way. Our time of prayer ended close to midnight but, instead of feeling more tired, Anthony and I had been refreshed by God's Spirit.

Miraculously I found that, by God's grace, I was still able to give, still able to serve other people. One evening Les and Jackie were talking about the possibility of sending an invitation to church at Easter to every home in the area. Within minutes I knew that I should write an Easter message and the words simply flowed into my mind and out through my pen. As the Sunday School Anniversary approached again the theme and content of the children's presentation became planted in me. As a result of that, I was asked to write a script for another Sunday School. I couldn't talk and couldn't 'do' much either, but God was using my love of the written word. Often I would have the feeling that I ought to write a letter to someone: again God's words would flow and his love would speak to them in their need.

One aspect of communication that I missed dreadfully was contact with children. Next door lived Jo's little boy, Matthew, aged three. He was wonderful: he would sit and chatter to me and didn't seem to mind that I couldn't reply, but I felt so inadequate. I wanted to chat to him too and show him that I was really interested in what he was doing. Then inspiration came. For his birthday I wrote him a book and illustrated it, called *Matthew's Dragon*. It seemed to be a point of contact that showed I cared. If I could do that for Matthew, I could do it for any child, and so ideas for stories teemed into my mind, each one designed for a particular child. It was an activity that fulfilled my desire for communication, and also delighted the receiver.

Our material needs continued to be met. By April I was finding it difficult to manipulate the clutch and gear lever in our car. What I needed was an automatic. Within days Anthony's uncle, who owned a garage, lent me an automatic car while we looked around for something suitable to buy.

When we did find the right car, the money was provided by two generous relatives. Meanwhile, food continued to flood in until we thought we would need a bigger fridge. One week we had eight sponges in the freezer because we couldn't keep pace with the influx. Offers of practical help in the house were numerous. My friends gave their services in this way with a lot of sensitivity. Lynn always gave the impression that her passion in life was to defrost a freezer, clean a kitchen floor or change a double duvet single-handed! Jo, with two young children to contend with, would regularly materialize beside the car just as I had returned from a journey—not really to see me up the path, of course! She would tell me she had 'time on her hands' so could she load the dishwasher or hang out the washing?

One morning in June, Sue, a friend from the village, called. She had something to ask me. Would Anthony and I mind if they called a prayer meeting for us in the village hall? I was overwhelmed. For months the vision of such a meeting had been in my mind, but I felt it would be selfish of me to suggest it to anyone. Yet, as the idea spread amongst friends and relatives, many said that it was a vision they shared also. The meeting was planned for 12 July at eight o'clock...

As I write the end of this particular chapter it is now 11 July. The response to being invited to the meeting has been amazing. Even mums that I met at the school gate who don't profess Christianity are keen to come along. I know God is going to move in a powerful and exciting way tomorrow evening. If, through that meeting, one person is led to Jesus, then I shall certainly praise God for the last eighteen months.

Chapter 10

WAITING BY THE
TELEPHONE

The weeks after the meeting were a period of both crisis and blessing. That evening Anthony and I prayed at home, and later we were joined by Sue and David and Lynn and David who had organized and led the meeting. They brought a huge card signed by everyone who had attended—a visual record of our friends' prayerful support. Over seventy people had crammed into a room in the village hall—believers and those not so sure, relatives and friends, even people not known to us personally.

To the accompaniment of the 'old tyme music' in the main hall, these people had prayed fervently, silently, tearfully for me and my family. The knowledge of their strong love and longing for us was a great source of encouragement. The meeting had been a special time for many people in different ways and I received letters from those who had found their own lives enriched.

Two images stand out in my mind as I recall that evening. One is of a normally effervescent friend who remained sitting alone at the end of the meeting with a stunned expression on her face. She said to another friend, 'I've never seen such faith!' Surely all the preaching in the world about faith cannot replace an actual demonstration of it.

The other poignant memory is of Anthony's cousin, Andrew, who went home from the meeting expecting the phone to ring and to hear me speaking. When the evening passed with no phone call he told his wife, 'She'll ring in the morning.' What faith! In recent months Anthony had felt drawn to a passage in the Bible where a sick woman touched the hem of Jesus' cloak, and Jesus turned to her with the wonderful words, 'My daughter, your faith has made you well.' As Andrew went on waiting by the telephone to hear my voice, so we also waited to hear the voice of Jesus speaking healing words to us.

Yet my physical condition continued to deteriorate, and this stirred up a terrible anguish in me. I felt as if I had been clinging on to the edge of a cliff by my fingertips, always believing that a line would be lowered and hoist me to the freedom and safety of the cliff top. There I would run, dance, embrace my family, sing, shout, scream for joy.

No rope was in sight. The shaly cliff was giving way and I felt that I was slipping beyond the reach of any lifeline.

Walking became so tortuously slow that even my car, my ticket to a little independence and freedom, became inaccessible. The gentle incline of the garden path seemed like Mount Everest. Also, not only did I now need lifting in and out of the bath, but I had to be helped out of the armchair. Every morning seemed like a night-mare: Anthony would hoist me up into a sitting position on the bed, help me to dress and then help me to stand. As I started to walk, my limbs felt as stiff as a tin soldier's and I had to lean forward to maintain my balance. Housework became a frustrating burden: just moving something from one place to another was a slow, painful exercise. It was evident that we needed extra help, and mechanical aids, in the home.

For months Dr Stevens, our family doctor, had been ready to enlist extra help. With sensitivity he recognized my stubbornness and pride and waited for me to give the go-ahead. With professionalism and tact he warded off the well-intentioned cries of those who seemed to think he should initiate help regardless of my feelings. One Tuesday morning in July we visited him at the surgery and requested a wheelchair, a home help and a visit from the health visitor to assess what other aids I might need.

I came home and broke my heart. I felt as if I had opened the floodgates to an army of official strangers, that I would be overwhelmed by all the trappings of disability. I had been forced to give in; surely now there could be no path back to physical wholeness. That morning I felt so wretched I prayed, 'Please, Lord, send me one of my close friends.' Five minutes later in walked Gillian, who listened, prayed and cheered me up.

During these days the hurt I felt inside was almost a physical pain. One evening Anthony hauled me out of the bath and seeing the grimace on my face said, 'There, that didn't hurt did it?' I pointed to my heart. 'Yes, I know,' he said, 'it hurts inside.' Anthony understood; he also knew the pain.

I grieved for my lost womanhood. I couldn't bear not fulfilling my role as a wife and mother. Sometimes late at night when everyone was sleeping I would make imaginary plans for the next day: I would get up early and have breakfast waiting on the table for the family. After dropping the children at school and a quick tidy round the house, I'd meet a friend in town. We'd have a browse round the shops and chat over a cup of coffee. On the way home I would pop into the supermarket for the week's groceries. Once home I'd phone my elderly aunt to make sure she was all right, and I'd take out a drink and cake to Anthony in the field. After school I'd take the children to the swimming pool and on the way we'd chat and tell silly 'Knock, knock' jokes. At bedtime, I'd tuck them up with a story and a cuddle. Anthony and I would share a quiet evening together and I'd tell him how much I love him...

I still grieved deeply for my voice: if I had to be so limited physically it would have been a great compensation to talk. I was given an additional machine which would 'speak' my typed-in messages in a voice that sounded like a dalek from Dr Who! Visitors marvelled at this £1,200-worth of equipment, but for a while I rather despised it. No machine could express the love, laughter, concern and encouragement I longed to give my family.

Progressive illness is not only cruel to the victim, it is equally cruel to the family. It was awful to see Anthony so tired doing all the things I should have been doing, to hear him shout at the children through sheer frustration, to see the pain in his eyes. It was awful to sense Claire's anger sometimes and Becca's frustration, feel powerless to diffuse the situation and comfort them. There were moments when I questioned the very meaning of salvation in my life: if I had been saved, what was I doing in hell? I felt rather disappointed with God and decided to keep my distance. I dreaded any visitors who might embark on Christian counselling and certainly didn't want any more prayers for healing—I'd been let down too often already, hadn't I?

What a good job that God's love and faithfulness to me doesn't waver like my love towards him. Despite my tiny mustard seed of faith, which seemed very small indeed, God continued to shower me with blessings and encouragement.

I dreaded the advent of the health visitor, fearing that she would herald a procession of strangers telling me what to do. In fact I was so churned up about it that I foolishly burst into tears as soon as she entered the house! But Sally was the opposite of all my fears and I soon regarded her as a friend. Her positive attitude and openness to self help was a great boost to me.

Sally introduced me to Sara, an occupational therapist, who also put no pressure on to accept aids that I didn't feel ready for but offered practical help in areas where I could regain some independence. An electric can-opener meant that I no longer had to send the children out to Anthony or our neighbours to open beans or cat food, extra rails on the stairs reduced the peril of scaling them when no one was around, and a special seat worked by compressed air helped me make a more dignified entrance to and exit from the bath. Sara also made us aware that a grant was possible for a downstairs bathroom, so we set about obtaining estimates and arranged a meeting with the Grants Officer.

Finding a chair that I could get out of was a problem: some didn't have enough power in their lifting device while others threatened to catapult me through the window. Our local branch of the MND Association got hold of just the right model—a chair which at the press of a button gently elevated me to a standing position. This provided the children with a new trick to play on unsuspecting visitors who sat in the chair. Suddenly they'd find themselves rising!

Another device which brought peace of mind to Anthony was the Tunstall Telecom System. If I fell or needed urgent help, I simply pressed a red button on a pendant round my neck; this would alert a central office in Truro who would then ensure that a neighbour called. Often when small children have been around the tempting red button has been pressed accidentally. Everyone treated these false alarms with good humour, seeing them as practice runs for the real emergency.

My wheelchair arrived with a dose of Christian fellowship. The delivery agent was a friend whom I hadn't seen for a while but who had been involved in prayers for me. His presence and conversation made the advent of the wheelchair less daunting—a sort of blessing on my new set of wheels. Claire and Rebecca were very excited about it and for the next few days everyone who came had to see 'Mummy's new chair'. If anything positive has come out of this illness for the children, it's that they will grow up with a healthy attitude to disability—neither afraid nor embarrassed.

I was granted a home help for an hour a day, but again had visions of a matronly soul taking over the running of the house. What a relief when I met Sylvia! She is a Christian and already knew about me through the prayer group of her church. Now Sylvia is like another member of the family; she doesn't just do her job, she gives us emotional and spiritual support as well. A heaven-sent home help.

One day, my friend Christine said that I really ought to have a word processor to help with all the writing I was doing. Ever since I had dabbled unsuccessfully in some computer studies in my sixth-form days at school, I had been very wary of anything along the lines of a computer, but Chris assured me that the word processor she had in mind was 'user-friendly'. Perhaps it would even smile at me? She also seemed to think that she could materialize one from somewhere; I was to ask no questions and leave it to her. Within days she returned with a processor and printer loaned by a mystery person for as long as required. With Christine's easy-to-follow instructions I discovered that indeed it was friendly, even to me. Now I spend so much time tapping away on the keyboard with one finger that I view it as a rather dear friend.

What had I learned, then, from these days with their mixture of dejection, encouragement and change? It was another friend, Lindsey, who helped me make sense of it. Lindsey had been a keen attender at the prayer meeting, which was something outside her previous experience. She pointed out to me how, although I had not been made physically whole again, I had received a lot of practical help that was widening my horizons. She set me thinking and now I try to praise God for anything that helps reopen a path that the disease has tried to bar me from.

Anthony and I are involved in constant combat with this disease. We dare not give up fighting for a moment. The apostle Paul used the vivid picture of Christians needing to put on the special armour that God has provided in order to fight evil. Every day we need to be in full battle dress!

Chapter 11
ODD SOCKS
AND COBBLESTONES

I cannot remember the exact day on which I took my last steps but during the last week in August walking was slow, painful and hazardous. Bent almost double to maintain balance, I leant heavily on my tripod with my right hand while grasping chairs, cupboards, walls and doors with my weak left hand. I was keenly aware that these were my last days of walking, but each faltering step was a protest against the relentless march of the disease.

One Sunday morning I was so determined to prepare dinner for the family that I stayed home from chapel. It took me an hour and a quarter to set the table for four, turn on vegetables already prepared and make some gravy. Afterwards I was too exhausted to eat any dinner!

With a huge sense of defeat we requested an electric wheelchair for use around the house. Acquiring one does involve a few yards of red tape, so while we waited I was given a chair with large back wheels so that I could propel myself manually. This was not ideal! While my right arm was strong enough to turn the right wheel, my left arm was too weak to manoeuvre the left. This would have been fine if I had wanted to turn in circles all day! For six weeks I was completely grounded, having to stay wherever I was put until Anthony could move me again. It meant deciding where I wanted to be for several hours at a stretch and ensuring that all I might need was at hand. If the tissue box was out of reach I'd have to sniff; if the television controls were out of range I'd have to put up with a programme I had no desire to watch; if I'd forgotten to request paper for the printer I sat frustrated, unable to complete a piece of work. It was frustrating but also claustrophobic: an awful sense of panic sets in when you are trapped in one place. When I was told that the wait for an electric wheelchair could be six months I became very depressed. If my days were numbered I didn't want to waste a minute being stuck somewhere wasting time.

Sylvia, my home help, decided to pray with me one morning—for a waiting-list miracle! It was a prayer answered in an unexpected way. The next Saturday morning we had a visit from Andrew, one of Anthony's cousins. He was armed with a tape measure which he wielded round me with a smug smile. At eight in the evening he returned with his brother, Nicholas, and another very tangible answer to prayer. There stood my big wheelchair with luxury attachments! All that afternoon Andrew, Nicholas and Nicholas' father-in-law, Douglas, had been working on its adaptation. By means of a battery, a windscreen-wiper motor, various wires, and two switches I was able to move effortlessly round the house again.

The next day Anthony and the children excitedly reported to all our visitors that Mummy set the table for dinner. Less than a year before this would have been an insignificant statement; now it was a triumphant proclamation!

There were two other features integrated into my new chariot—a very resonant bell and a GTI badge! The bell was a great substitute for shouting at the children and a way of getting my own back on Anthony when he teased me! The chair became a neighbourhood attraction and when my doctor made his regular visit it was very amusing to see him and Anthony extolling the mechanics of the chair and virtually ignoring me. This made me feel very normal! My response to them for their ingenuity and to God for answered prayer found expression in a light-hearted but heartfelt poem of thanks which I presented to each of them:

Ode to Andrew, Nicholas and Douglas

I was stuck in the pits, frustrated and sad,
I had wheels but no propulsion,
'Til three engineers with angels' wings
Had an ingenious notion.

First Andrew arrived to measure me up—
Had me worried for a while!—
But the surprise he brought back
Soon revived my smile!

Into my life there came a new friend—
A souped-up wheelchair
That whirred and moved and gave me legs—
A tangible answer to prayer.

The team had adapted bits from cars
With ingenuity by the ton.
Then added an L-plate, a GTI badge
And a deafening bell for fun!

So now I'm on the road again
But I'll pull in to give a hug
To my three engineers with angels' wings—
Andrew, Nicholas and Doug!

Three weeks later I received a visit from the gentleman who has the power to allocate electric wheelchairs. My previous impatient thoughts towards him completely faded when I realized that he alone was responsible for wheelchair allocation for Plymouth, Cornwall and the Isles of Scilly. No wonder the waiting list stretched to six months! Again my souped-up chair was a source of amusement and interest. Of course in his official capacity he hadn't really seen it, but he proceeded to request a demonstration! He then announced that as I had demonstrated satisfactory handling of the chair I could be allocated an official one quite quickly without the usual test drive.

Apparently before letting people loose with these chairs they have to ensure that they won't endanger themselves, the family or the house. I could understand why when my electric chair arrived less than a week later. The steering is extremely light, so that at first I constantly threatened the paintwork, furniture and family feet! Also the speed is adjustable and, as Anthony remarked, when it's at full power you have to be able-bodied to cope! The children think it's a great joke to adjust the speed when I'm not looking so that a slight touch of the joystick sends me hurtling forwards or back! There are just two things missing—a bell and a badge.

When I was able to walk or even limp but not to speak, many people shouted as though I was deaf. Now that I'm in a wheelchair and unable to speak many people presume I can't think. I can understand this reaction, but it still hurts. Tradesmen sometimes get edgy: unsure of my state of mind and wary of my attempts at communication, they chat heartily to anyone but me and make a relieved, hasty exit. A young mobile hairdresser felt timid: she anxiously asked friends how bad I was and after postponing two appointments lost her nerve completely. One friend who pushed me out for a breath of fresh air adopted the indulgent tones and pram-peering actions of a new granny! Even the most well-meaning people can touch a sensitive nerve, such as the dear friend who likes to refer to me as 'her invalid' and compare me to her frail mother who is well over eighty!

The advent of the wheelchair was also a signal for

well-intentioned troops to invade our home and take over. Things done out of pure kindness and generosity can seem suffocating and threatening. People waltzed into the house without ringing the bell; sometimes two people at one time would be upstairs sifting through our clothes, gathering washing and reorganizing cupboards; the fridge overflowed with stews, pasties, pies and desserts. As a result we had more food than we could eat, a pile of odd socks and an overwhelming feeling of superfluousness.

Some restraints were called for! Anthony replaced the leaky washing machine with a new one and claimed exclusive rights to the washing; a meal rota reduced the food mountain; and learning to postpone visitors sometimes afforded us space to just be a family. If it were a short-term illness, no doubt I would have sat back and enjoyed others 'getting on with it', but knowing that my inactivity was to be a permanent feature, there surfaced in me an instinctive desire to protect my territory! I felt like a jealously protective lioness!

Life in a wheelchair does have its funny side. Our first outing was on August Bank Holiday to Porthleven, a delightful Cornish fishing village with an excellent ice cream parlour. Unfortunately another feature, previously unnoticed, is its drainage system! Sometimes high winds whip the water over the harbour wall, so every few yards a wide-open drainage channel cuts through the pavement so water can run back into the harbour. This meant that every ten yards the front wheels of the chair lunged into a dip, leaving me gripping the sides to avoid sliding out! The alternative to this checkered route round the harbour was to hog the narrow road. It was then I really discovered that so-called quaint villages owe much of their charm to unstructured roads! Every bone and joint appreciated that charm and quaintness; the girls cushioned me with their cardigans and Anthony muttered something about shock absorbers!

One rather touching feature of this maiden wheelchair push was Rebecca's constant presence at my side like some angelic guardian! She held on to the arm as if it were my hand and with a gleaming face entered into the new experience with great enthusiasm, even pride.

There are three people who regularly take me out. Each has their own peculiar style and each has a special place in my star-award scheme! Points can be scored in two sections: transfer skills and pushing prowess. My friend Christine takes me shopping each week; she scores highly on both sections. Anthony says it's because she's used to horses! Certainly she approaches the whole operation with the calculating mind of a point-to-pointer and handles this sensitive creature with a great deal of strength! Together we have discovered the hassles involved in shopping with a wheelchair. The first obstacle is the heavy swing doors that threaten to catapult us on to the street again before we've man-oeuvred inside. Worse are steps which completely bar my entry; here Chris occasionally parks me outside and darts in and out with an assortment of items for me to choose. Once inside, narrow aisles are often a nuisance, especially in my favourite bookshops: we endanger merchandise and other customers, and browsing is out of the question! Shopping has to be planned around the large modern stores with lifts or the single-storey shops.

Truro is a beautiful city which has preserved many of its cobbled streets, a feature that adds another dimension to wheelchair riding! We bump and shake along the street until I raise a hand to signal stop and Chris repositions my feet which have vibrated off the foot-plate! Despite these hazards Chris always makes shopping seem effortless and fun; sometimes we get a fit of the giggles and I have to suppress my dreadful hyena-sounding laugh before too many people stare!

Lynn, who approaches the whole of life with

wholehearted enthusiasm, attacks taking me out with similar verve! I will say little about her transfer skills except that sometimes between the car door and the seat there doesn't seem enough room for her, me, the chair and her enthusiasm! If we start laughing I am in serious danger of missing the car seat completely!

If there were speed limits for wheelchairs Lynn would be heavily fined. We charge from shop to shop and if the pavements are too crowded we take to the road, defying any oncoming traffic! No obstacle diverts Lynn from her goal: one day when searching for a special-occasion dress Lynn was determined to get me inside a shop with several steep steps, so she collared an assistant and hijacked a passerby and together they hauled me and the chair into the shop! Another time we attended a coffee morning at a friend's tiny cottage. The front door was just wide enough to admit the wheelchair but it was impossible to squeeze through the interior doorway. Again Lynn marshalled the troops and I was swiftly transferred to an ordinary chair before being carried sedan-fashion into the main room!

Anthony, like most men, has an aversion to shops and shopping, so most of his stars are won or lost on the transfer section of my award scheme! It is a standing joke that when a physiotherapist enquired which method my husband uses to lift me I replied, 'The same way he lifts the other livestock on the farm!' Anthony has to transfer me from bed to bathroom, from wheelchair to easy chair, in and out of cars and chapel pews and up and down the stairs, so if sometimes these operations lack dignity I don't complain. Most of the time I feel very safe and Anthony knows he has a very special place on my star chart!

The arrival of the wheelchair heralded the demise of my car. This was a tremendous disappointment because it meant that all my hopes of taking the children to school were dashed and a rota of lifts had to be drawn up. It was painful to see even my close friend, Gillian, taking them off to school at the beginning of the September term, especially when Claire had a fit of colly-wobbles at the thought of her first day in the Juniors.

I was their Mum; I should have been taking them to school. I should have been reassuring Claire and giving them both a hug at the school gate... This miserable disease continued to rob me of my children's lives. Guessing how I would be feeling, Lindsey called round at nine with a fistful of tissues and some excellent cheering-up lines! Apparently, mums or no mums, half Claire's class had made a sobbing, anxious entrance that morning!

Anthony promised to take me to meet the girls from school on Tuesdays and Thursdays. Besides just wanting to be there for them, I'm far too inquisitive to miss out on the 'gathering of the mums' at the school gate! That first afternoon was the first time most of them had seen me in a wheelchair. Towards the end of the previous term so many of them had attended the village prayer meeting to pray fervently for my healing, and here I was now so obviously worse. I admit to wanting to apologize on God's behalf, to say how sorry I was that their mustard seed of faith had not been honoured...

At that moment I desperately wanted to get up and leap around, not for myself but for them. I wanted to demonstrate God's power to answer prayer in a way they could instantly recognize. How presumptuous of me! Two months later I was to learn how powerfully God could move through my weakness and because of my disabilities.

Chapter 12
WE'RE OFF TO SEE THE DUCHESS

Although late Summer heralded the next stage in my physical deterioration, it also sparked off a series of events that were exciting, encouraging and which satisfied a lifelong ambition. They confirmed that were I, by a miracle, to regain my voice, the word 'coincidence' would never escape my lips!

Each month as I trundled through the supermarket checkout with my trolley full of groceries I used to grab a copy of the magazine *Family Circle*. One of the first articles I would turn to was Dee Remmington's 'Winning Through' series: there, in a thoroughly honest and unsentimental manner, people related how they coped with and overcame difficult situations that affected them and their families. As far as I knew the subject of a terminal illness hadn't been tackled and from early July I had an increasingly insistent compulsion to write to the editor: to congratulate them on the series, to suggest they tackled terminal illness, and to outline how we coped with Motor Neurone Disease. For a while I tried to dismiss the idea—I wasn't in the habit of writing to papers or magazines and I was nervous of sounding patronizing, or, worse still, attracting sympathy for myself. The idea, however, wouldn't go away so one Monday in late July I sat at the typewriter: 'Dear Ms Churchill, As a regular subscriber to *Family*

Circle...'

The words flowed through two-and-a-half pages... 'I am writing this not to gain sympathy, which is a negative reaction, but to engender empathy. Yours sincerely, Jenny Richards.' The letter was launched into the post-box together with a prayer—'Lord, direct and use this letter as you want.' He certainly did!

One Friday about three weeks later, a letter arrived from *Family Circle*. They explained how my letter had landed on their desk on the very day they were starting plans for an article on Motor Neurone Disease. They had in fact been writing to the Duchess of York, who is patron of the Motor Neurone Disease Association, and so had forwarded my letter to her. Coincidence...?! They said they would be contacting me again soon. 'Soon' was the following Monday. I could hardly believe what was happening when they rang to ask if two people from their Features department could come down from London on the following day to interview me!

Deborah Murdoch and Helen Travis arrived at two on Tuesday afternoon and spent three hours with us. It marked the beginning of a friendship that stretched beyond the bounds of the article. I shall always appreciate their sensitive approach to the interview: they recognized the pain involved in relating harrowing events and occasionally joined me in reaching for the tissues. It was also an exciting experience for me: journalism had always captured my interest, so I was fascinated to learn that in August they were preparing for February's issue and that within a few days they would be tucking into the Christmas fare prepared by the Cookery department for their December issue.

Before leaving they confronted us with a thrilling proposition: would we all like to attend the Motor Neurone Disease Association's Annual Conference at the National Exhibition Centre in Birmingham and be presented to the Duchess of York? If so, *Family Circle* would meet all our expenses. Needless to say we were very keen. Our only concern was how Anthony could cope with the children as well as me on such an expedition. The problem was quickly solved: Anthony's mum, always game for an adventure, offered herself and Anthony's dad as itinerant childminders! During the next few weeks Deborah was frequently on the phone making the necessary arrangements:she even ensured that the hotel was prepared to cater for my boring but established eating habits! It wasn't often they received requests for mashed potato followed by yoghurt.

About a week later the postman delivered a registered letter—postmarked Balmoral Castle. Imagine my excitement when I discovered that the Duchess of York had sent me a three-paged letter in her own handwriting. It was very moving to sense her genuine concern for our situation, to read her words of encouragement and to learn of her prayerful desire to work towards the conquest of the disease. The style of her letter lacked any trappings of formality: it was written as one friend to another, as one mum to another. For a week friends called—not to see me, but 'The Letter'. Everyone was touched by its warmth. For days the children sang, 'We're off to see the Duchess, the wonderful Duchess of York!' to the Wizard of Oz tune.

On Thursday 14 September we set off from Truro on a five-hour train journey to Birmingham. Thanks to *Family Circle* we travelled first class. While it afforded us more space, it also made us more aware of the pitch and volume of the children's voices! It was good to have Granny and Grandpa around, not only as another source of amusement for the girls, but also to help with disembarkation. To land me, the wheelchair, my machine, cases and children on a bustling platform, and keep us moving in the same direction was no mean feat! The efficiency of the station master was impressive: I was listed among three wheelchair passengers whom he was expecting and, although he seemed rather agitated that one was missing, he ensured we surfaced safely from the station and despatched us in a taxi to our hotel.

The hotel was ideal—spacious with good facilities but comfortable enough not to worry about every sound the children made. I kept thinking what fun it would have been if I was well: swimming with Anthony, Granny and the children, instead of merely spectating through a window; sitting in the rarefied atmosphere of the dining room midst sparkling glasses and shining cutlery, browsing through a tall, glossy menu, savouring at leisure a meal that had variety, texture, taste. Of course, had I been able to do all this, we wouldn't have been there.

We woke on the Friday morning with a colony of butterflies in our tummies. Anthony took great care to ensure that his three girls stayed in pristine condition and then spattered bacon fat on his own suit. We arrived at the National Exhibition Centre at ten o'clock and, although the Duchess wasn't due until lunch time, there was plenty to keep us occupied. Naturally *Family Circle*, one of the sponsors of the conference, wanted to report the event in a forthcoming issue, so as soon as we had met up with Deborah and the photographer we had to go outside and re-enter the building so it could be captured on film! We also had to be reintroduced to Peter Cardy, the Director of the Motor Neurone Disease Association. I think we both felt a fraction silly nodding and smiling at each other while the camera rolled.

I felt sorry for the photographer who had been landed with us as his subjects: Anthony was camera-shy; Claire, when nervous, tended to scowl; Becca liked showing off and my mouth muscles were so weak that when I tried to smile I looked as if I was in pain. It couldn't have been one of his easier assignments.

The Duchess' schedule was running half an hour late and the children began to get restless: Becca rolled under the table with 'Blanket', her ragged comforter, and

Claire wanted to go back to the hotel for a swim. Eventually word came that Her Royal Highness was in the building, at which point Becca decided she desperately needed the toilet. Granny discreetly rushed her there and back.

At last the Duchess started to make her way round the huge conference room. I was concentrating on keeping my composure: as I have mentioned, MND makes one's inner emotions very visible—not only twinges of sadness, but also joy and gratitude can reduce me to tears in seconds, and I didn' t want it to happen as I shook hands with the Duchess. I think having to use my machine helped—it gave me something else to concentrate on. All week I had been tapping useful sentences into its memory such as, 'Good afternoon, Your Royal Highness. It's a pleasure to meet you.' And, 'Thank you for your letter. It was very much appreciated.'

Now at last Peter Cardy introduced us; the Duchess' black-gloved hand reached forward and I tapped out my greeting. The warmth exuded in her letter was instantly recognizable as she chatted with us: earlier that week she had announced that her second child was expected, so I congratulated her and she asked us if having two girls was good. Claire, usually the shy one, kept tugging Anthony's arm. When, after several tugs, there was no response, she pushed forward and addressed the Duchess directly—'What are you going to call your new baby?' The Duchess explained that she hadn't decided yet!

Before moving on she told us to keep strong. This was no flippant farewell gesture—they were the words of someone whose patronage of the Association had been born out of a close friend's struggle with the disease. She was keenly aware of the endurance called for in both sufferer and carer.

It was this identification with families affected by the disease that characterized her speech to the conference.

As part of that speech she quoted from my letter to *Family Circle*. As she read, tears welled up in Anthony's eyes and Claire and Rebecca burst into loud sobs. I was aware that they moved towards the back and that Deborah placed a supportive hand on my shoulder: I can only put it down to a mini-miracle that I managed to grit my teeth and stop my face from crumpling.

While the Duchess completed her address, my family were being rescued by Mr Geoffrey Dear, the Chief Constable of the West Midlands Police: indeed one of Claire's fondest memories of the trip is wearing the Chief Constable's smart braided hat! His concern and kindness was the hallmark of everyone we met at the conference. The children's tears clearly upset the Duchess who returned to us to make sure we were all right. For a few moments we were the ones reassuring her and I found myself typing out 'Don't worry' on my machine.

The press were far more daunting than the Duchess and as soon as she moved on they surrounded us. 'What did your little girl ask?'...'What did the Duchess say?'...Anthony even had to give a short interview for the local radio station. We awaited the morning papers with a little trepidation.

After such an exciting and emotional occasion, it was refreshing to attend two short, informal talks on Nutrition and Physiotherapy. It was also an opportunity to meet fellow-sufferers—although, as one gentleman pointed out, fellow-copers is a better expression. Two things were evident: the disease seemed to affect more young men than young women, and the progress of the disease varied significantly. There was the ex-army officer who had run the 1989 London Marathon: a week later he had difficulty running one hundred yards; a month later he needed a wheelchair. Yet there was another man who after seven years had limited use of his hands but only a slight slurring of speech and slight walking difficulties. It also surprised me to observe the kind of food others were eating—things I hadn't been able to eat for months. On more than one occasion during the conference I found myself looking at someone with obvious handicaps and thinking, 'Poor chap, how dreadful for him!' and then realizing that I was no better. I know that I am severely handicapped but I don't perceive myself as handicapped. Much of this I owe to my friends who have continued to treat me as the same person I've always been.

During Saturday's breakfast time the papers arrived. There on the front page of *The Birmingham Post* was a headline that rather shook me—TEARS FOR A DYING MUM. Again, although I knew I had a terminal illness, I didn't label myself as dying: each day I aimed at living, at achieving something, creating something. The three papers reporting the Duchess' visit milked to the full this sentimental side of Friday's events, and, although I found it unnerving, I had to hope that it would alert more people to join the fight against MND.

Saturday was the main day of the Conference and the place teemed with people. There were lectures, workshops, exhibitions, entertainment, but my most vivid memories of the day were the people I met: Peter Cardy and his colleagues who, despite the pressures of organizing the event, made time to chat and displayed the friendliness and concern of an extended family; a delightful elderly gentleman called Geoffrey whose words 'God bless you' carried an almost tangible strength; so many strangers who introduced themselves and wished us well. Before leaving home I had wondered if the Conference would be depressing. It wasn't. I left with an even greater desire to fight, not just for me, but for every coper, carer and association worker and member I had met. As we left the National Exhibition Centre they were tears of sheer emotional exhaustion, not depression, that poured down my face.

On Sunday we had a long journey home in a train

with a buffet car but no staff to run it. For once my own little store of mousses and yoghurts was a coveted feast.

Coming home was in no way an anticlimax, for in the next few weeks some really exciting developments took place. With the support and guidance of the staff of *Family Circle* I realized my lifetime's ambition of having some of my writing published. Ever since they had sampled some of my work in August they had been generous in their encouragement and keen to link me to a publisher. Now they offered to use two pieces of work in their own magazine—an adult short story and a children's story. I was actually in print. It seemed incongruous in a way that, while so much of my life was closing down, here was a longed-for career opening up.

I was continually conscious of God's loving purposes for me, and very much in mind of some words of Jesus: 'I have come to bring you life in its fulness.' He certainly wasn't allowing MND to cheat me of that vital gift: despite physical deterioration, there always seemed to be another adventure round the corner.

Chapter 13
PREACHING WITH
NO VOICE

Nearly a year had passed since Sunday 23 October 1988, when I had felt God calling me to preach again. I had done all I could to answer that call by embarking on the preachers' training scheme in the Methodist Church. Part of that training was to lead Sunday worship regularly, with Anthony as my voice. As I had become more disabled, it was difficult to fulfil these preaching appointments. Anthony had more and more responsibilities in the home and it wasn't fair to burden him with yet another duty. In August 1989 I had had to pull out of the scheme. This was a terrific blow that shook my faith: had God really called me, or had it been just my own wishful thinking? If he had called me, why was he closing the door in my face so soon? For weeks these questions tangled in my mind. For a while they affected my attitude to prayer and church attendance: how could I be sure which voice was God's?

One Monday evening I got an answer. The phone rang and Anthony answered. After a short conversation, he came into the room saying he hoped he had done the right thing. Apparently one of the County's Methodist Youth Leaders had asked if I would speak about my faith at a National Youth Rally at St Austell. Anthony had said no, thinking that it would be too much for me to cope with emotionally. But in my mind there was no hesitation: I felt as if God was standing right beside me saying, 'I've called you to preach, I've called you to preach!' I knew that I had to say yes and let God look after the physical and emotional difficulties.

When Anthony rang back to say that I would speak, we learned that over two thousand young people would be there. God had certainly confirmed my calling in style. A lot of my friends considered me crazy: Lynn stood in the kitchen, hands on hips, declaring, 'You're mad!' but, as Anthony and I pointed out, at least my knees couldn't knock nor my voice shake!

Two weeks before the rally, Stephen Emery Wright, an effervescent young American minister, called to plan exactly how I would speak. I volunteered a friend, Christine Roberts, to be my interpreter: besides being a preacher and youth leader, she had also taken over my last teaching post. We decided that the guest speaker, Peter Crewe, would ask me a series of questions: What is MND? How do you cope? How does God use you? What about the future? Chris would stand by my side and read out my answers from a typed sheet.

As I sat at the word processor to prepare my answers I was given a very clear vision of the message I had to get across to those young people who were gathering from all over the country. I had to tell them that Jesus makes all the difference to our lives, that despite all the awful things we might encounter in life, nothing can separate us from God's love and care. I felt totally inadequate to deliver this message—how ever would I have the emotional strength? I had to launch myself completely on the ocean of God's power and let him carry me and my words in the direction he chose. I know Chris felt the same: she had to trust God to stop her knees knocking and to protect her emotionally too.

So it was that on Sunday 22 October 1989, exactly a year after my call to preach, Anthony wheeled me into the Cornwall Coliseum, the county's largest venue. The building vibrated with noise and colour: a rock group pounded on the stage, while young people clad in green and yellow sweatshirts and scarves stamped, clapped, shouted, chanted and hugged each other. This service was the culmination of a hectic weekend's activities: they had tackled mini-assault courses in the rain, discovered Cornish pasties, struck up new friendships, slept on hard schoolroom floors. The atmosphere was charged with excitement and anticipation.

Just as impressive as the noise was the silence that descended blanket-like when the service began. A white-clothed figure carried a huge cross on to the platform and a voice read out a 'loveletter' from God. There were hymns, greetings, readings, a dramatic presentation of the relevance of the Cross in today's world, and then it was us! There was no ramp on to the stage, so Anthony and Stephen had to haul me and my chair up the steps and leave me to Chris' steering. We emerged through the curtain and were immediately relieved to find that the dazzling spotlights prevented us from seeing more than the front few rows.

As soon as Peter started chatting to me I began to feel at ease and to feel the thrill of being able to communicate with young people again. 'How old are you?' he asked. 'Ancient!' I tapped out. He asked me about my machine and I demonstrated its dalek voice. Then the main interview began. As Chris read out my answers I didn't feel sad, embarrassed or cheated: I was so sure that it was a special message from God that it didn't matter who spoke it as long as it was heard. When we turned to leave the platform people stood and clapped: at that moment I felt as if I would burst with the sensation of God's strength filling my weak and totally inadequate shell. I also wanted to stand and clap God for what he had said and done. Never before had I felt so humbled, so uplifted.

God spoke to many people that morning. During the

last hymn a youth leader from Sheffield came to me, and tearfully described how God had spoken to him and members of his youth group during my testimony. There were many others who searched me out and gave me a hug that said it all.

Outside the rain had cleared and we posed for photos in bright sunshine. The event was to be reported in the *Methodist Recorder*, a magazine for Methodists which is distributed both in this country and abroad. I was amazed, though, to discover that my testimony had been printed in its entirety. The letters I received from readers confirmed that this was a message God wanted to be heard, and I had to face some inescapable questions—would God have been able to use me so effectively if I hadn't been ill? Should I even be thankful that I hadn't been healed if it meant that, through my disabilities, God was calling people to a greater level of faith?

I also thought back to the prophecy that I had received over a year before when the preacher had declared three things: that I shouldn't worry about a reduced income; that I would preach to thousands; that my health would be restored. The first two had now been fulfilled. Why shouldn't the third part come to fruition? Surely it was no more difficult for God to heal me than to use my dumb, disabled body to preach? Facing up to these questions involved me in thinking through the words of that hymn that I had received in the early days of my illness. The last verse began:

'Take my will and make it Thine,
It shall be no longer mine...'

Abandoning one's self completely to God's will is not easy. It involves saying, 'Right, Lord, if you can use me more effectively in illness than in health, in death than in life, then so be it. I am completely happy about the situation.' I haven't reached such heights of faith. Surrendering my will to God's will is a daily struggle.

My calling to preach, even without a voice, continued to be confirmed: all I needed was God's inspiration, which never failed, a workable right hand and my dear friend, the word processor. I was asked to write an article for another Christian magazine. Again I was deeply moved by the response of the readers who wrote to me explaining how God had spoken to them, and encouraging me in my quest for greater faith. Local churches also requested contributions for their magazines.

In September our church had a new minister who started visiting me regularly and, despite the fact that he had not known me in my pre-MND days, we soon struck up a good rapport. One day he asked if I would write services for people called 'Readers' to deliver in various chapels in our area. I was delighted. I was beginning to understand how God wanted to use me. With every sermon and article I wrote I felt strengthened inside. Very familiar Bible passages took on a new significance for me. A good example is Psalm 23—a psalm often recited as a panacea for all ills and in danger of tripping off the tongue with little attention to its real message.

'The Lord is my Shepherd;
   I have everything I need.
He lets me rest in fields of green grass
   and leads me to quiet pools of fresh water.
He gives me new strength.
He guides me in the right paths,
   as he has promised.
Even if I go through the deepest darkness,
   I will not be afraid, Lord,
   for you are with me,
Your shepherd's rod and staff protect me.'

This picture of God as a shepherd was now a daily

reality to me. He wasn't the modern shepherd who rounds up his sheep from a distance, but the shepherd of the Psalmist's day who walked ahead of his flock, the first to encounter the danger, and always looking for the finest pastures.

Despite the decay in my body, God continued to lead me into new and thrilling experiences, to green grass and fresh water. Time after time he gave me new strength: I could recall numerous occasions when I had felt defeated and had questioned the purpose of going on fighting the disease. Then I would find myself challenged by a new project and feel a sense of purpose and enthusiasm flowing into me again. These new challenges were surely the 'right paths' referred to in the Psalm. I was acquainted with 'the deepest darkness' and knew that in human terms it could become even darker, but I also knew the care of the shepherd who led the way, clearing a safe pathway with his rod and snatching me from danger with his crook.

When my illness had first been diagnosed my Aunty Barbara told me that she would pray that I would be 'protected'. At the time this puzzled me, but gradually I realized how God was constantly answering that prayer. In physical terms I was living a nightmare and yet there were so many positive opportunities for me to grasp and enjoy. I believe the Good Shepherd protected me from much of the horror of my situation.

Chapter 14
'TIS THE SEASON TO BE MERRY

Each year from mid-November onwards the world seems gripped in a frenzy which we like to call Christmas. Television advertisers scream at our children with the latest toys; the town is full of worried, scurrying shoppers who spend plastic money as if there's no such word as 'debt' in January. In supermarkets obese trolleys jam the aisles while people grab siege-like quantities of food; the media serenade us with sentimental songs and assure us that if we toss in a few pounds to 'Feed the world', then we can sit back and 'Have yourself a merry little Christmas.'

Everywhere people ask one another, 'Are you ready for Christmas?' 'Well, I've bought all the presents; now I must ice the cake and I'll be ready.' Ready for what? In recent years I've become increasingly aware that we spend a great deal of energy and money preparing for Xmas, but little or no time preparing for Christmas. Xmas is the celebration of 'X', the unknown quantity; Christmas is the celebration of Christ, God's special gift to the world.

It isn't that I want to abolish the colour, the lights, the parties, the presents. I enjoy all these traditions. There are times, though, when the compulsive drive to create a merry Christmas can cause pain and distress. As one good friend remarked, we like to play happy families even when it may not be possible or appropriate. This was my experience of Christmas 1989: I wanted to give presents, send cards and letters, spend time with Anthony and the children, but I also longed to run away from all the sentimentality of Christmas.

December 1989 marked the end of the two years I had been given to live: I was on bonus time and grateful for it, but further signs of deterioration indicated that I wouldn't be around for another Christmas. My neck and back muscles weakened: sometimes my head would fall backwards and I would experience a dreadful choking sensation until someone rescued me. Dressing had added complications because I could no longer perch on the edge of the bed—I kept flopping backwards and sideways like a limp rag doll. The most distressing deterioration, though, was in my right arm and hand: gradually the fingers were curling, the wrist stiffening, the upper arm losing its lifting power. Eating and drinking became exhausting activities as I struggled to manipulate and lift my fork or cup. A half-full plastic cup of tea took the best part of an hour to drink. With characteristic stubbornness I resisted Anthony's offers to feed me.

It also meant that writing became difficult: I wrote with the unsteady deliberation of a four-year-old and signing my name on cheques in shops became an embarrassment. One day I had to send a specimen signature to *Family Circle* for use in the article. I cried with frustration as I tried to get it right. Losing my signature was a further loss of identity—a little bit more of me was disappearing. Until now I'd never realized how often I scratched my head or ear or nose. It is extremely irritating not being able to reach an itch, and extremely demeaning to ask someone else to do it for you!

With this as a backdrop to Christmas, I wrote a poem and submitted it to our village magazine. I discovered that I was not alone in my quest for a Christmas in which we become more conscious of Christ.

Follow the Shepherd Boy

One clear night a shepherd boy, dazzled by stars,
Hurried to a stable and found the fulfilment of his
forefathers' dreams.
Returning to the hillside, his heart sang with new
hope for the world.
Today, dazzled by neon lights and persuasive
advertising,
We hurry to the shopping centre to fill trolleys
chin-high.
Plastic money quivers in the frenzy of a vampire
Christmas
Until credit hangs like an albatross around the neck.

I want to escape!
Take my hand, shepherd boy—lead me to the stable.
Let me clasp the hands of others seeking refuge,
comfort, hope...
The child from Beirut, the hostage from Lebanon,
The earthquake victim, the starving child,
The unemployed father, the dying mother...
Show me a key to unravel the world's insanity.

I look up—
High above the baby's head two rafters cross—
God has kissed the world with his gift of love!

I run back to the crazed shopping centre.
I want to slam shut the tills, silence the advertisers'
clamour...
I want to shout and scream in the streets,
'God loved the world so much he gave his Son...
Follow the shepherd boy...he'll show you!'

And watch, as politicians, terrorists, rulers, church
   leaders,
You, me,
Journey to that stable,
And, dazzled by a cross of love,
Discover the Gift who will change the world.

My world was certainly changing. Although in many
ways it was telescoping as further deterioration imposed
more limitations on my ability to do certain things, in
other ways it broadened as I was presented with new
opportunities. A lifetime's ambition was realized when it
was agreed that this book would be published. As I
discussed publication and worked on the final chapters I
was given a great sense of purpose and employment. It
was a great boost to morale to sit at the word processor
each day, knowing that my writing now had an assured
goal. It was the kind of fulfilment I used to feel when
teaching something to children who grasped it with
enthusiasm and imagination, and it was so good to
experience that kind of fulfilment again.

I also created and fell in love with a penguin! Rebecca
was fascinated by penguins and for well over a year I had
been wanting to write a story about one. As we lived in
the village of Perranwell, I thought Perran would be a
good name for him. One November day I was inspired
by an idea: I would write a collection of stories about
Perran the Penguin centred round the local school;
children at the school could do the illustrations; it could
then be printed and sold for school funds.

Here at last was something I could do for my children's school. I so hated not being able to help with
swimming, library duties, outings and fund-raising
events. The idea was received with tremendous enthusiasm and I derived a great sense of fun from this
project, not only in creating the stories but in meeting
with other mums and the printer, and in sifting through

the children's wonderful drawings. One evening our sitting-room was carpeted with a hundred penguin pictures!

For me this creative activity was a further sign of God pouring his love into me. My body was wasting but the real me—my mind, my spirit—was constantly being revitalized.

People continued to be vital channels of God's love, and often in unexpected situations. One day I had a visit from an occupational therapist who moulded me a splint to encourage my fingers to straighten. She noticed the children's Sunday School leaflets on the table and started asking about the church we attended. She was also a Christian and asked if I would mind her praying with me! Since then Maureen has joined the ranks of my many caring friends.

One Friday evening Anthony phoned the printer to make some initial enquiries about the penguin book. He was a friend of friends so we had occasionally met at parties. Later Vivien explained the significance of that phone call. For months he had been praying for me but recently had a growing conviction to visit me and pray with me. He was hesitating—after all, he didn't know me well and he wasn't in the habit of bursting in on people and declaring he had come to pray. On the Friday of the phone call he should have been away but the trip was cancelled at the last minute. When he heard Anthony's voice he knew he had to risk any embarrassment and come. Viv is a quiet, gentle, sensitive person, and as he read from the Bible and prayed with us, he communicated these aspects of God's nature. I knew God understood everything about me and that in my suffering he was constantly in me and all around me, encouraging me, protecting me.

Being unable to do so many things means that small, ordinary things take on a new significance. I love it when one of the children perches on my lap; when they rush in from school and excitedly share their news with me or perform for me a new rhyme or recorder piece. In pre-MND days Claire and I used to enjoy getting messy in the kitchen making sticky iced buns and oozing jam tarts, so when she asked me to help her make some buns for the Brownies' party it was a special moment. I sat in the kitchen typing out instructions while Claire successfully coped with weighing and mixing. I had discovered an activity we could still share and it really thrilled me.

At the end of term the girls were involved in school plays: Rebecca was uncharacteristically a mouse in *Little Red Riding Hood* while Claire was a singer in the Nativity play. I attended the matinee with some trepidation: I was conscious that this could be my last chance to see them perform and I worked hard at maintaining emotional poise. I knew that one touching expression could tap the well of tears that trembled just beneath the surface. Rebecca decided to show off by swinging her mouse's tail round and grinning impishly at the audience. Claire, however, having acknowledged our presence with a half-smile, approached her role with seriousness.It was indicative of how each child dealt with life in general: Claire—thoughtful, sensitive, easily hurt; Becca—bouncy and undaunted. How I loved them with their differences! I didn't cry: *Little Red Riding Hood* made me laugh and the innovative approach to the Nativity play was totally absorbing.

During November and December there were some changes in the house. For three weeks builders and plumbers moved in and converted the playroom-cum-dumping ground into a spacious toilet and shower room and separate office area. People moan about builders but apart from the inevitable layer of dust that settled throughout the house I rather enjoyed their cheerful company. I was constantly serenaded by two who had wonderful voices. The downstairs bathroom made certain areas of life much easier: Anthony had to haul me upstairs only once a day and sitting under a shower took the precariousness out of bathtime. The office area was cosy and bright, a delightful room to work at my writing.

A week after the builders left, the possum arrived. This is not a stray Australian creature but an ingenious machine which enables me to control my environment. The engineer arrived with several boxes of equipment and metres of wire: with the help of my brother-in-law, an electrician, he ran wires under carpets, through cupboards and along walls. Then he attached a computer-like screen to the wall and gave me a little black box to hold. By pressing lightly on the box a list of words appeared on the screen; when I pressed again each item illuminated in turn: if I wanted to call Anthony I would wait for the word 'alarm' to light up and set it off by taking my hand off the box. In this way I could open the door, pick up the telephone, switch on lights, the television and the radio. A little independence at my fingertips.

On Christmas Eve Anthony received a most unwelcome gift—a vicious flu virus. I had never seen him as ill as he was in those next two weeks. Our traditional Christmas had already been eroded by my illness; now it completely disintegrated. The children spent most of the holiday with relatives and friends and, although I was grateful for this hospitality, I missed them. During this time I felt very depressed. I sat and watched Anthony breathlessly struggling to look after himself and me. I lay helpless while he became exhausted trying to dress me; I dangled awkwardly in his arms as he battled to climb the stairs.

Over ten years before we had vowed to love and cherish each other in sickness and in health: Anthony had been fulfilling that promise relentlessly; now, when he needed some extra special cherishing, I was useless. I ached to take care of him, to wrap him up with a hot water bottle, bring him hot drinks, keep the fire going, keep the children amused and let him sleep long and deeply. At the same time it was frightening to realize how much I depended on Anthony. He was the only person who fully understood how MND affected me: what food was palatable; the right position for sleeping; my topsy-turvy emotions; so many little idiosyncrasies. He was the only person who understood some of my words without using my lightwriter. Always he brought tremendous positiveness to our situation, constantly encouraging me.

People often tell me I'm brave: three-quarters of that bravery is down to Anthony. While he had the flu I realized more keenly than ever how my well-being was inextricably linked to his. Although he would never admit it, this utter dependability must be an awful burden, a burden which with all my heart I wish he'd never had to carry.

That was Christmas 1989. If I am no longer around for Christmas 1990, at least the family won't be able to look back to the previous year with any sentimental longing. If, however, my condition should arrest or miraculously improve, may Christmas 1990 be one to recall with thankfulness.

Chapter 15
'...AND A HAPPY NEW YEAR'

Most people begin the year by making resolutions; I began 1990 by tapping out my last wishes. During my illness Anthony and I had avoided talking about death, not because we were afraid to face facts, but because we believed that concentrating on life was the only way to cope with the disease. Knowing that my right hand—my talking hand—was failing, I felt compelled to share my thoughts with Anthony while I was still able to communicate adequately. Anthony had always teased me about being organized—I used to delight in planning events and working through copious check-lists. I have approached my own funeral in a similar way although I can't be sure of the date and time.

I want it to be a celebration of the life God has given me and of the love I've shared with family and friends, so I have chosen hymns that reflect these things. The first hymn will begin, 'Oh for a thousand tongues to sing my great Redeemer's praise...' For two years I have longed for my tongue to be released; I have often cried in church or when listening to tapes of worship songs because I was unable to vocalize the joy I felt inside. When they sing those words at my funeral I shall be joining in: I shall be free of the shackles of MND; my spirit will sing and dance.

Besides discussing the practicalities of the funeral and

97

burial, I wanted to assure Anthony that he must feel free to marry again: he and the girls deserve a 'good woman' to look after them. Sometimes I wish I could choose someone and hand the three of them over with references. MND's cruellest blow is to deprive me of my family. I grew up knowing the pleasures of family life and feeling so secure in the love that surrounded me. It is this pleasure, security and love I wanted to share with my husband and children. Talking to Anthony in this way felt unreal; it was as if I was listening to someone else. Surely it wasn't Jenny Richards, aged thirty-five, having to say these things?

During the first week in January the flu bug decided to visit me. Although I wasn't as badly affected as Anthony had been, it brought me to a crisis point in my illness. I lost a lot more weight which could not be replaced by my limited diet. I appealed to my doctor, 'Can you do something to keep me going for two months so I can finish my book?' Within two days he returned with the solution—a jejunostomy. In layman's terms, this involves inserting a tube into part of the digestive system and feeding liquid food through the tube. It obviously involved an operation and a stay in hospital which filled me with dread. I had never been operated on before so there was fear of the unknown, but, even worse, was the thought of being in a strange environment with people who didn't know me and might not understand my illness. I had a fortnight to wait.

It was at this point that I could no longer struggle to feed myself and had to face the indignity of being spoon-fed. The disease was stripping me of every ounce of independence. One Friday morning, at an all-time low, I tapped out a message to my friend Lindsey, 'I'm failing and I'm a coward.' Later she returned with a letter expressing things that were too charged with emotion to say aloud. Her letter was as strengthening as a three-course meal. She said how much she valued our friendship, how through my illness I had helped others appreciate life, and then she recalled an occasion in pre-MND days when we had laughed together. 'That,' she wrote, 'is how I will always remember you.' Too often embarrassment prevents us expressing our love towards people: then, when it's too late, we have regrets.

Until January I had said that there was no physical pain with MND. This changed with my additional weight loss. Sitting all day became extremely uncomfortable and staying comfortable at night was an impossibility. Rebecca's brightly-coloured swimming ring was the answer in the daytime. I perched on it like a huge bird waiting for something to hatch—in fact it became known as 'Mummy's nest'! The nights, though, continued to be nightmares. Three or four times I would wake with pain in my shoulder, my neck or my legs and Anthony would have to move me. This interruption of sleep made it increasingly difficult for him to cope and, in Anthony's words, 'we hit a wall'. We had to enlist more help. Again, the speed with which people swung into action was impressive: sitters stayed with me for four nights, giving Anthony the chance to catch up on much-needed sleep; the MacMillan nursing officer brought a special mattress which made the bed more comfortable and a team of three district nurses called regularly to shower me and wash my hair.

On the Thursday before my stay in hospital the phone rang. 'Is that Mr Anthony Richards?' an American voice enquired. It was Khris, my penfriend, from Michigan. We had been corresponding for twenty-five years but had never spoken. She had been so upset to hear of my deterioration she had felt compelled to express her feelings and to pray with us. As she prayed and Anthony and I linked hands it seemed as if the three of us were in the same room. There was a tangible sense of God's love holding us tightly together despite the miles between us. Khris and I had shared an ambition to meet one day, when our children were grown up and we were more free to travel. Anthony has a plan: when the miracle happens and I get better, we will fly to Michigan. A fantasy? Maybe, but whenever I'm in danger of giving up Anthony reminds me of Michigan. It is our password for keeping positive.

On the morning I was due to go into hospital Claire decided to allay any fears by playing shrilly on her recorder and singing a made-up song about how I'd be all right, there was nothing to worry about and I would be home again soon. I think she felt her cheering-up plan was in jeopardy when Becca announced with relish, 'They are going to cut Mummy's insides with a knife!'

On arrival at the hospital, I was relieved to find I had a single room. Despite my interest in people, I couldn't have faced being in a ward with other patients and unable to communicate freely with them. That morning we were seen by various staff: all were understanding in their approach but none had previously encountered MND. This made me feel rather insecure and I dreaded Anthony leaving me. I could identify with the small child clinging to the parent with whom he feels completely safe. My main worry was that I would find myself in a situation where my head was lying flat and I'd be unable to communicate that I was choking. I therefore proceeded to tell everyone who entered my room about the need to keep my head raised.

When Anthony did leave, panic set in. It suddenly dawned on me that I was on the Chest Ward—why? Then the physiotherapist came, encouraging me to breathe deeply and assuring me that she would be on hand after the operation to help me. I knew that MND affected the muscles controlling breathing but not until then did I recognize my own inability to sustain deep breaths. My mind reeled: what if the anaesthetic adversely affected my breathing? What if I came round fighting for breath? Was there a risk involved that no one had told me about? If I was able to walk I would have discharged myself. When Anthony returned for evening visiting I poured out all my fears: he must make some enquiries and if there was any risk get me out before the operation the next day. Never had I felt so frightened, so trapped. It was a well-timed visit made by Elspeth, the MacMillan representative in the hospital. Into my panic she poured her quiet confidence and dispelled much of my fear. What remained was the natural anxiety of anyone contemplating an operation for the first time.

The day of the operation lingers in my mind in a series of impressions: the clinical smell of the medicated bath; a fond farewell to an unscarred stomach; the regulation white gown and funny hat; waiting; turning pages without reading; the inevitable call to theatre; the horizontal journey down squeaky-clean corridors; the dry humour of the anaesthetist; the opening of the theatre doors, then—nothing; the realization of being alive and breathing; the unaccountable passage of time...

For almost a week afterwards I questioned the wisdom of my decision to have the operation and frequently regretted it. My only food was through a drip and I felt weak, helpless, bored and misled. When eventually I was allowed to start feeding through the tube it took ten hours to pump through the contents of one 500ml bottle. I envisaged being attached to a machine for the rest of my life. In fact, I felt very unlovely: how could Anthony find anything attractive about a wife who needed wheels to move, a machine to speak, a computer to write and now an ugly tube protruding from her stomach? Constantly Anthony reassured me; constantly I grieved for the life that he was losing because of my illness; he didn't deserve me.

I was salvaged from becoming completely drowned in negativity by a tremendous tide of love that flowed through many channels: Gillian's daily letter; the flowers that transformed my room into the semblance of

101

a florist's shop; the cards that covered every available surface; the loan of Becca's toy kitten to keep me company; Claire's grown-up assurances that I was looking better; nurses like Vidhya who, also in her thirties with two children, listened to me and encouraged me; Irene who constantly made me laugh with her special brand of humour. As the feeds increased and took less time to be pumped through it was Irene who nicknamed me 'Miss Piggy' and blamed me for her bad back.

During my second week in hospital *Family Circle* published their February issue, which included the article about us and our meeting with the Duchess of York. It was quite alarming to flick through the pages and be confronted with our own faces. But we were delighted with the sensitive treatment of our story. Nurses dived off to lunch breaks with a copy; relatives and friends rushed to the shops until, within a week, Truro had sold out! The most rewarding aspect was when people said that they now understood a little bit more about what it's like to have MND. The article had achieved its goal.

Coming home was almost as strange as going into hospital. Foolishly I expected to feel different immediately. Instead, new routines, a procession of visits from medical personnel and some potent sleeping tablets made me listless and rather dejected. Again, it was only the strength of love that helped me see beyond those bleak, windswept January days. A very touching example is a letter I received from a twelve-year-old girl called Anna who had read an article I wrote for a church magazine. She wrote:

'It is marvellous what God has done for you, and the love that people have given you. Please give my love to your family. I will be praying for you, and I will be praying that you will live.'

The love and depth of feeling in those lines was a source of strength and hope.

When I attended Grammar School the last activity of each term was to cram into the school hall for a final assembly. Always the Deputy Head stood at the lectern and read the same lesson, 'I may be able to speak the languages of men and even of angels, but if I have no love, my speech is no more than a noisy gong or clanging cymbal...' For years those words were synonymous with the release and freedom experienced at the start of a school holiday. Now when I read that Bible passage I recognize a different kind of freedom: it is about the love that has so frequently lifted me beyond the grimness of my physical condition. This is how Paul describes it in the rest of that passage:

> *'Love is patient and kind; it is not jealous or conceited or proud; love is not ill-mannered or selfish or irritable; love does not keep a record of wrongs; love is not happy with evil, but is happy with the truth. Love never gives up; and its faith, hope, and patience never fail.'*

I am constantly surrounded by family and friends whose love towards me is cameoed in this passage. 'Love is eternal,' says Paul. My Motor Neurone Disease will be conquered: one day it will be banished by a miracle, a sudden medical breakthrough or in death. The love I've received will never leave me—it will enrich my spirit for ever.

Chapter 16
THE FUTURE

It is now February 1990 and, according to the original prognosis, my time is up. I wonder how much bonus time I will be granted. Looking even a few months ahead can be frightening. This book is due to be published in six months' time. 'Great!' people say, 'That's not long.' But six months in the clutches of Motor Neurone Disease is the difference between speech and dumbness, walking and wheelchair confinement, an arm that can stretch high in the air and an arm that is unable to lift a tissue to a salivating mouth. It is the difference between breathing easily and being deprived of breath.

When I started this book I wrote in longhand; by chapter nine I welcomed the light touch of the word processor keyboard; now my hand gropes across even those keys like a lame spider—it has taken an hour to type out the last ten lines, and now I need to rest.

This recent deterioration is causing me to panic: my right hand is my only link between the me inside and other people—through it I express the stories, poetry, questions, laughter, love and anguish that would otherwise be trapped inside this limp, dumb body. My mind teems with new ideas, fresh projects: can I acquire the technology to communicate them? Can I acquire the time? Sometimes I feel as if I am trapped in a runaway train that will inevitably crash into the terminus.

Yet, what is the future? Does it really exist for any of us? Before my illness I used to plan for the future as if it was a concrete certainty: now I am learning that the only time we can be sure of is the present moment. As our minister said, we are all terminal—some of us just seem more terminal than others! How much do we miss by failing to savour today instead of worrying about tomorrow?

Today is the first day of the half-term holiday: while Claire went to market with Anthony, Rebecca and I spent the morning together at home. We watched a video; then played a board game in which Becca made the moves for both of us. She talked and giggled incessantly, her brown eyes wide with the excitement of living, her mouth almost permanently an impish grin. I caught her infectious zest for life and realized that it was good to be sharing these special 'now' moments with her. If I had dwelt on a future that might separate us, I would have missed the riches of our relationship today.

Maybe this is what Jesus meant when he urged his followers not to worry about tomorrow. He wants us to live each day with a positive attitude, grasping and savouring the good things we experience. This is why I aim to offer each 'now' moment to him so that he can fill it with his life. Each day I ask him to help me achieve three main goals: firstly to communicate my love to my family; secondly to help someone, maybe by sending a letter, maybe by listening; thirdly to create something, usually story-writing, poetry or sermon preparation. His life takes the place of my lifelessness and he continues to give me the strength and enthusiasm to meet new challenges.

Yesterday evening I attended a service at Kea Church where I had been invited to speak. Physically and emotionally it was a marathon: we arrived in time for the prayer fellowship at six and didn't leave until half past eight. During this time I had sat in front of a full congregation while my friend, Maureen, read my words, and afterwards had met and chatted to lots of friends, old and new. Medically speaking I should be totally exhausted today—indeed I was prepared for a relapse. Instead it's just the opposite: I feel stronger than I have for weeks!

Yesterday God was at work in two ways: as he used me to bring his love to the people at Kea, so he also used them to bring his love to me. After the service had finished a group of five people expressed a desire to pray with me. As Maureen voiced her prayer, she became hesitant, almost afraid to speak aloud the vision the Lord had given her, for it was a picture of me standing. As an occupational therapist she knew that it was medically impossible: she appealed to Bob, the vicar, 'I don't know how to pray.' He then prayed that I would be given the ability to stand spiritually, and, if it was God's will, to stand physically. Today I have indeed stood spiritually: I have felt a great joy and peace welling up from deep inside. Physically also I have experienced renewed energy. I dare not contemplate complete healing—I am savouring today's little improvement.

My next challenge is to speak at a school assembly at a local girls' High School. They are raising money for the MNDA and want an insight into the disease. It is exciting to be able to communicate with young people again, and I marvel at the way God continues to provide opportunities for me to do things that bring me fulfilment.

I used to sing a chorus with these words: 'For me to live is Christ, to die is gain.' I am increasingly aware that without Christ my life is meaningless. So much of the me that other people saw has disappeared: the busy mum, the housewife, teacher, the chairman of this, the secretary of that. Even my personal appearance has changed. Last week I was confronted by my reflection in a full-length mirror and I did not like what I saw: I was slumped awkwardly in the chair, my legs and feet swollen and misshapen; my clothes clung and gaped in the wrong places; my hair lacked bounce, the parting too defined; my face, weakened by muscle wastage, looked too long and sad, and saliva dribbled down my chin. Only Christ can create a new life out of the ashes of my previous lifestyle; only he can create beauty from the distortion of my body; only he can bring laughter bubbling out of a blank expression. Perhaps this metamorphosis is the miracle of healing...

'...to die is gain.' This is where I struggle. I love life and the little girl inside me stamps her foot and screams at God—'Daddy, I don't want to die!' I ache to watch Claire and Rebecca grow up, even if it is a silent vigil. I long to share more of life with Anthony. I would like to grow old with friends and reminisce about the 90s! Yet I know that when I die I shall experience even more of the love that God has showered on me in life.

Sometimes I play a fanciful game: if I could regain three experiences before I die, which would I choose? I toy with several ideas: to squat on the floor by the fire, munching hot buttered toast; to relax in a hot, deep bubbly bath; to make and eat a Cornish pasty; to phone a friend. Always, though, I return to the same three choices. I would walk on the cold, smooth sand at the water's edge and feel the tiny, icy waves tickling my toes. I would sit on the bed with the children, an arm round each one, and read them a story. I would throw my arms round Anthony and hug him so tightly.

During my illness I have gained fresh insight into many situations: into the frustration of a small child who lacks the words to communicate his needs; into the anguish of an old person struggling to maintain independence and yet hampered by a slowing body; into the painful emotions of a person coming to terms with his total dependency on other people. Above all, though, I have gained a fresh view of God's unfailing love. In the Bible Paul writes:

'Who, then, can separate us from the love of Christ?
Can trouble do it, or hardship or persecution or hunger
or poverty or danger or death?...No, in all these things
we have complete victory through him who loved
us...there is nothing in all creation that will ever be able
to separate us from the love of God which is ours through
Christ Jesus our Lord.'

These words are a daily reality to me. It is this experience of God's love that makes the difference between being terminally ill and terminally blessed.

Some plants, such as lavender, release powerful perfume when they are crushed. I like to think that out of my life and the lives of my family, crushed by Motor Neurone Disease, there might have emerged something positive. Maybe we've been able to help in a small way to heighten people's awareness of the disease and bring the cure a little closer. Maybe we've helped someone appreciate the life they had taken for granted. Maybe, through our attempts to express our faith, God has touched someone in a special way.

The following lines are my testimony to the triumph of God's love.

> I try to speak a word of love—but make only ugly
>   sounds,
> I try to caress—but my hand is crippled and
>   ungiving,
> I try to complete a loving deed—but my feet are
>   heavy and slow.
> Inside my heart breaks—out flood guilt, grief,
>   anger, disappointment.
> The stench and ugliness of disease are all around.
> Self crumbles...

But look!...
In the selfless place a miracle occurs.
A broken voice finds new expression,
Crippled hands, slow feet, move in a new dimension.
In and out of the broken heart flows a healing tide of
   love,
From the crushed ruins of self rises a sweet
   perfume...
It is the aroma of Christ—
Fragrance of my living, fragrance of my dying.

N.B. Jenny died on Christmas Day 1990. Her condition had remained unchanged up to a week or so before, when she experienced considerable extra pain. The doctors were called to the family home on Christmas Eve. Jenny was given pain relief, went to sleep and never woke again - - - - -

"Then shall I see, and hear and know

All I desired or wished below

And every power find sweet employ

In that eternal world of joy."

HALLELUJAH!   P.43.

THE RESPONSE TO JENNY'S 'WINNING THROUGH' FEATURE

When *Family Circle* ran the feature on Jenny in their February 1990 issue (see Chapter 15), many readers responded. Most contributed to an appeal for the Motor Neurone Disease Association; many wrote of their feelings. Here are a few quotations from their letters. (The writers have all agreed to being quoted.)

Dear Family Circle
I've just shouted at my two sons, the kitchen is a mess, and I've had a row with my husband. Then I read Jenny's story. Today really is wonderful. Please find my cheque enclosed.
Yours
Mrs J. from Hampshire

Dear Editor
I have just read your article 'Jenny's Story'. It was so heart-rending I couldn't stop the tears, and yet Jenny Richards' bravery absolutely shone through. I wondered if I could be so courageous as Jenny Richards if the same ever befell me.
I fervently pray that some time in the near future the mystery to this disease will be unlocked and a cure be found, or even better, prevention.
Yours sincerely
Mrs S. of Lichfield

Dear Sirs

I was extremely moved by your article about Jenny Richards and her very courageous attitude to life. All mothers must wonder sometimes what would happen if they should become very ill and then push this dread to the back of their minds and pray that it does not happen to them. Your article showed that illness can strike anybody and that we should all live our lives to the full and enjoy every moment of our children's lives.

Yours faithfully
Mrs I. of Kidderminster

Dear Family Circle

I read the letter from the brave woman Jenny this morning...I am now going to fill my days with plenty to do, and live life to the full instead of wasting the precious little time we all have on this earth.

Yours
Miss C. from Kent

Dear Editor

After reading your article in the magazine about Jenny, I showed it to our Head Teacher and said that as Jenny was an ex head girl of the then Grammar School we should do something to help your appeal. During the last week of our term, the P.E. Department had planned an Active Health Week, so I approached them to see if it was possible to make a grand finale to the week and get the whole school involved in a Sponsored Fancy Dress Fun Run. Extracts of the Family Circle article were read to all students through assemblies and they were all asked to take part. Many of our students were very moved by the article and set about earnestly collecting donations to run. A large notice board in school read:

CAN YOU RUN?
JENNY CAN'T
RUN FOR MOTOR NEURONE DISEASE

The money we will donate to the local MND Association in Cornwall, so that Cornish sufferers in particular can be helped directly.

Yours sincerely

Mrs D., principal pastoral teacher at Camborne School

Dear Family Circle

As I lay in the bath last night reading Jenny Richards' story, I cried for her courage and her spirit 'still dancing'.

My two children are the same age as hers and when the youngest was only two my husband suffered two heart attacks at the age of 31. I am ever thankful that he made a complete recovery, but we will never again take the happiness and good fortune we share for granted. God bless her, I know I will think of and pray for her often.

Yours sincerely

Mrs S. of Orpington

Dear Family Circle

This evening I read your article on Motor Neurone Disease, and was deeply touched. Two years ago my family and I were involved in a horrendous car accident that left my husband and I badly injured. I often feel very, very depressed at the prospect of a future of never-ending and worsening pain and disability. Thank you for making me see how fortunate I am, to have even limited and painful mobility.

Please send my heartfelt respect to Jenny, and fond regards to her brave husband and daughters. You have made me personally much happier and more able to cope, through your heartbreaking story. Thank you Jenny.

Yours very sincerely

Mrs B. from Sussex